Understanding Psychological Evaluation and Treatment: Donny's Story

TABLE OF CONTENTS

INTRODUCTION   1

SECTION I: Evaluation and Intake

               Psychoeducational Evaluation

               Intake Evaluation for Possible Therapeutic Treatment

SECTION II: Rational Emotive Behavioral Therapy (REBT)

               History of the Founder

               Construct of Personality

               Human Thinking from the REBT Perspective

               Example of Therapeutic Sessions

               References

SECTION III: Adlerian Therapy

               History of the Founder

               Construct of Personality

               Techniques and Procedures

               Twelve Stages of Adlerian Therapy

               Example of Therapeutic Sessions

               References

SECTION IV: Existential Therapy

               History of Founders

               Approaches to Existentialism

               Major Constructs

               Existential Concepts

               Concept of Therapy

               The Therapeutic Process

    Examples of Therapeutic Sessions

        References

CONCLUSION

APPENDICES

    Appendix A: Intake and Suicidal Risk Assessment

    Appendix B REBT Worksheets

    Appendix C Adlerian Therapy Worksheets

    Appendix D Existential Therapy Worksheets

Dedication

This book is dedicated to Donald Francis Kimball, whom without, there would be no story. This will forever be part of your legacy. We are indebted to you. This book is also dedicated to Jeffrey M. Carboni who had his own struggles in life. May this book help those who are touched by those who are suffering internally, so that they can reach for the help that they need.

INTRODUCTION

Born a fiery red head, Donny was the first child of Lee and Gerry Kimball. Lee, raised with an Irish and Jewish influence, and Gerry, raised with an Italian influence, Donny was no exception to the feisty traditions of his heritage.

After 36 hours of delivery, Donny appeared in the world with a large head, a bruised left side, and his left eye swollen shut. On the same side of his head, he sported a cauliflower ear. His hands and feet were huge in proportion to his body.

Food allergies soon surfaced and led to irritability as a baby, with long nights and colic type problems. Allergy shots were soon to come to the rescue. However, he did not like the shots, and liked even less that his mother was the person from whom they were administered.

Gross motor capabilities were never in question. By Christmas time, at the age of 7 months, Donny was escaping from his crib. He could even scale a book case, and at one point, the daredevil that he was, he toppled a one onto himself. These moments never seemed to disturb his constant motion. He simply powered on.

At times, he even escaped the house, leading to an incident where he freed himself from the apartment, and to the horror of his mother, toppled down a flight of stairs. But when she picked him up at the bottom he was delighted by the experience and said "gin, gin." He was ready to repeat the experiment. True to his nature, undaunted by the experience, his adventurous spirit continued. Parental requests to slow down and be more careful were ignored.

A job offer in California took the couple away from extended family, into a quaint town where neighbors would soon adopt the couple as family. Such neighbors, and a close babysitter, had the opportunity to see the unique qualities of an agile young child who could "climb tall buildings in a single bound."

In one such bounding feat, his babysitter Connie told the following story:

"I remember him climbing this huge tree. He must have been 70 feet up. In my surprise I said, 'Donny, what are you doing up there? Get down or you'll break your neck.' I don't know how he even got up there. The bottom branches were at least 10 or 20 feet off the ground."

And his apparent super hero like climbing habits were by no means confined to trees. He also liked roofs. One neighbor, who would soon be known as Grandpa Bill remembers the following experience with Donny:

"One day I found him sitting on the very highest point of my garage roof. He was about five years old at the time. Where he was sitting was at least 15 feet above the ground. Not wanting to startle him, I nonchalantly greeted him and asked what he was doing up there. He said he had climbed up to pet our cat. I asked if he had, he said 'no' – the cat had 'took off' when he approached it. But he said it was 'fun' to be on the roof anyway. I asked him if he could get down okay. He replied 'oh yes' – that he had done it many times, and he proceeded to scramble down using a patio cover support to make it the last few feet to the ground. As gently as I could, I told him it was not safe to climb on the roof and asked him not to do it again. He said 'okay.'" To Grandpa Bill's knowledge he respected that wish, as he was never found by the Richardson's on the roof again.

Nelson, another neighbor, witnessed Donny's climbing habits and remembers:

"During the time that he and his family lived across the alley from us, I was remodeling the house next door. Often, Donny would come over to see how things were going. He was very agile and seemed to enjoy climbing up the wall to the attic crawl hole which was ten feet above the floor. He did not use the ladder. In the adjacent room there was a hole through the floor to the basement. One day, at about dusk, Donny came over and did his usual climb. When he jumped down, he disappeared through the hole in the floor, much to the surprise of all of us. He was not hurt, but surprised, and I am sure his ego was jolted. He did not cry and kept a stiff upper lip."

Had YouTube been a thing at the time, Donny would have been an overnight sensation. His lack of fear and his curious nature would have brought the followers from all over the globe.

School was always a challenge for Donny. As early as preschool it was noted that he did not take naps and some of his fine motor skills weren't developing as expected. For instance, he could not tie his shoe laces. As he progressed through the educational system, his reading and writing were not developing at the same rate as his peers, soon to be determined that dyslexia would be his constant companion.

Often labeled a bad child due to tantrums that he would display both at home and in school, a keen Psychologist expressed concern over the possibility that these "tantrums" were actually seizure activity. Followed up by the neurologist, it was soon determined that this "bad child" was actually displaying seizures, something only medication could help.

Donny's Kindergarten teacher, a strict and often off the book's woman, set a classroom tone that Donny, a rambunctious child, did not fit into. One experience that highlights this was during an art class, where Donny painted in black and white. The teacher, being strict in nature, told him he had to use color. Not being a part of his plan, and after much nudging on her part to change his painting, he proceeded to throw the paint he was using. As this and other stubborn behaviors were disruptive to this teacher's idea of how a classroom should run, she notified the parents in an end of the year conference that Donny needed "a classroom for children who were mentally retarded." Psychological testing indicated that Donny was a bright and engaging child, that also struggled with Dyslexia and ADHD, making a typical classroom a challenge, and an educational setting with children with low IQ's an inappropriate placement. Thus began the long and discouraging journey with the educational system in California.

Despite his experience with his Kindergarten teacher, Donny did well in an ungraded summer school program designed to support his transition into first grade. Although he enjoyed summer school, first grade reinforced that the educational system was an undesirable environment for him. After a few weeks of attending, he started hiding under his bed and holding onto bedframes for dear life in an attempt to stave away the start of school.

Although he did not enjoy his learning environment, he did enjoy gaining knowledge. He was a confident youngster when it came to all things mechanical, although his experimentation with fixing things did not always end well. One day, after school, Donny crossed the alley with his 3-year-old sister in tow. He was headed out to fix a car. He proceeded to pour anything he could find into the neighbor's gas tank, including dirt, sticks, and various 'lost things' along the path. When they returned, Susan told her mom all about how he had fixed the car, already highlighting his mechanical curiosity.

By second grade, the school had determined that Donny would need more support in order to keep up with his peers, so once a day he was bussed from his neighborhood school to another grade school in the district to get special instruction. His curriculum focused on reading and writing skills. While making little progress with reading, his handwriting and math saw improvement throughout the year. However, the frustration of school still led to disruptive outbursts. It was noted that Donny tended to boil over with frustration before letting it all go, so his teachers also worked to help him identify his emotions and incorporate strategies to allow him to improve his behavior.

About this time, due to a lazy eye, Donny underwent tests to determine how that was affecting his vision, and if it contributing to his Dyslexia. This courageous fiery redhead had no concerns about having tests run, or going through surgery to fix his eye. He was more concerned about how much his peer's made fun of how it looked. Between his inability to keep up with peers, and the appearance of the lazy eye, he was becoming more aware of his fading self-esteem.

Despite these concerns, Donny made friends easily. By second grade he had a best friend, Charley, whom he played with on a regular basis. Charlie was fascinated with going to Donny's house. He had a tree house there that he worked on regularly, repairing it, changing it, whatever suited Donny's fancy at the time. His parents were wonderful about allowing him to do so.

Donny's determination, along with his curiosity and lack of fear made him a popular kid. Charlie remembered that one day he decided to chop down a tree in the backyard, so he went and got an axe out of the garage and made quick work of it. This lack of fear of parental consequences amazed his friends on a regular basis. Donny did not act out as a form of disrespect towards his parents, he loved his family very much. He simply did not fear their response.

By the time that Donny entered 4th grade, it was clear that a full day of school was asking a bit much. Donny's family had just relocated to the Greater Boston Area, and the schools there seemed better able to deal with a student that did not fit the typical classroom profile. They approved a schedule for Donny that brought him into the school for two hours of classwork a day, and then allowed him to be home perusing active learning for the rest of the day. This new level or responsibility worked well for Donny. He was able to explore the world around him in ways that were hands on and active. As this new schedule continued, his leadership abilities were able to shine through in his everyday interactions with peers. This level of independence suited him.

Although Donny loved his freedom, from time to time his parents worried about it. Saturdays were often stressful for them, as he would disappear for hours on end since there was no school or church to attend. His parents decided to enroll him in a YMCA program. However, the rigidity of the schedule did not allow him to vent his energy, and his outbursts began to escalate again. Eventually, his Saturday adventures were returned to him.

Another concern for his parents was his limited physical interactions with others. He rarely engaged in a hug or other displays of affection with his loved ones. In fact, it seemed to disrupt something in his senses if he did. At first, there were concerns about his ability to attach. However, during his time in Boston he had both a parakeet and a snake that he cared for and loved very much.

Donny and his family returned to Claremont, CA, in 6th grade, as his father's two-year work assignment was over. Upon return, the school system scheduled Donny for two hours a day of learning assistance. They did not, however, agree that Donny could be released from a full day of attending school.

The school psychologist completed a re-evaluation and noted poor impulse control and poor self-esteem. A full day of school did not suite Donny. To him, it was a return to a restrictive setting and he had no problem letting his teachers and other school authorities know his displeasure. He would often disrupt the class, yell at the teacher, and then walk out. As things escalated, his parents determined that he needed a break from the typical educational setting. They pulled him from school and allowed him to go work on a family farm for some time. His mechanical inclinations and leadership qualities were suited for a day of work outdoors. Upon return to school his behavior escalated again, and his school work did not progress, so it was decided that he would repeat 6th grade.

When Donny was informed that he would not move on to Junior High with the rest of his friends, he withdrew, was sulky, and would spend hours in his room or in the garage where he could tinker with all things mechanical.

As Donny returned to the 6th grade, the school noted that a typical day would simply render the same results that they had seen the year before, so they tailored a program that allowed him to go to the local high school in the afternoon and take welding. Donny was allowed to ride his bike about a mile to the High School. He was free again and gaining his independence back. His mood improved and he began to make older friends at the high school level.

Even though school was becoming more and more difficult, his mechanical abilities were thriving. His old babysitter gave him a 56 Chevy to work on during his free time. It was kept in the garage so he could go out and work on it whenever he had time. A neighbor gave him a mechanics book that had both pictures and text. Although he could not follow the written text, he was able to look at the pictures to work on the car. Donny identified a problem with the distributor. When he was finished fixing it, the car still did not start, so a friend took a look and noticed that it was wired "backwards." He let Donny know. Once Donny rewired the distributor the car hummed like she was ready to hit the road. There was always a question as to whether his Dyslexia played a role in his reversal of the wiring.

Donny was never shy on entrepreneurial abilities. In his new found independence, he passed through a park daily where the "pot heads" hung out. He most likely made friends with a few of them, allowing for experimentation of new mindsets. This assumption of his family was fueled by the fact that it was discovered that he was growing pot on the roof of the house.

At the high school level, Donny was taking welding and mechanics courses. His welding teacher was very impressed with Donny's skills. He was also acutely aware of Donny's disabilities, and decided to give him his exams orally. When he gave him his final exam, he noted that Donny had retained virtually all the information from the class. He received an A from the teacher, who noted that Donny was able to create sculptures with his welding tools. His parents were extremely impressed with his artistic aptitude in welding. At the age of 13, Donny was set up with an oxygen and acetylene tank, connecting hoses and several tips. This allowed him to create many works of art as an outlet to the frustrations that were building up due to his basic classes in school.

Donny, in his wisdom, determined that the tanks were also useful for experimentation. He began to fill balloons with acetylene and oxygen. He would then ignite the end of the balloon and run. The result was, for Donny, a very satisfactory boom! He continued to work on that until he got the perfect mixture, which would rattle the windows in the nearby houses. As all the neighbors knew him, they were quite tolerant of this behavior. His friends loved the effect, and served to solidify his reputation for having no fear. Despite Donny's reputation, he did not have a propensity toward criminal behavior.

At the age of 13, Donny began school at the local Jr. High. At El Roble, learning support was provided at the request of the student. They would simply drop into the classroom for assistance when they needed it. Donny chose to continue to utilize the help. It was noted by the support teacher that he could read better than half of the students enrolled in the program. He was offered the opportunity to enroll full-time in the learning assistance program, but his math teacher felt that he could handle the regular classroom, if teachers reached out to him and built rapport. The learning assistance teacher agreed. During 7th grade Donny was able to pass all of his classes with the help of the school and an at home tutor.

Donny continued to suffer from migraines which would keep him in bed for their duration. This was odd only from the perspective that Donny was usually found in motion, unless he was forced into a desk.

Eighth grade continued much the same, with the exception that he was now enrolled full time in the learning assistance program. He still required extra help, which he received at home through private tutors.

As a reward for working so hard during his Jr. High career, Donny was allowed to go visit his maternal grandfather for the summer. A proclaimed mountain man, and true to his Irish heritage, his lifestyle was right up Donny's alley. Their days were filled with hunting and roaming the woods of upstate New York, in particular the Adirondack Mountains, which his grandfather knew so well. The afternoons were filled with time at the local bar where he would enjoy the story telling of his grandfather's cronies. Donny was taught how to drive in the backwoods that summer, and also learned the game of darts. As a reward at the end of the summer, he was sent home with one of his grandfather's .22 rifles, with the expectation that as Donny returned for hunting expeditions, he would become the owner of his grandfather's prized riffle collection.

Donny returned home to a rigorous application for a High School that was known for its mechanical program. In fact, if students remained in the program for 5 years, they would leave with both a High School Diploma and an Associates of Arts Degree in mechanics. As they progressed through the program, they would receive various mechanical certifications along the way. But the Academy had very strict admission requirements. At first glance of his grades, they felt that they were unable to admit him. However, with the intervention of a family friend, it was determined that he would be granted a space at the school under certain conditions. They labelled Donny a special student so that he could take any class in the Academy. However, to graduate he had to maintain a 2.0 grade average in his academics. The committee provided Donny a special circumstance request to take oral exams instead of written one's, but in Donny's desire to be seen as "normal," he rarely exercised this option.

Initially, Donny's grades were promising, carrying a 2.2 grade average coming out of his first semester at Don Bosco Technical Academy. As he was keeping up with his school work, a family friend suggested the possibility of Donny working part-time at a local gas station. In doing this, he would be offered the ability to apprentice as a mechanic. Donny thrived in this situation. His employer noted his aptitude. Along with being trained as a mechanic Donny pumped gas for full-service clientele. One of Donny's closest friends who worked with him, noted that Donny often struggled to fill out the forms.

During the summer between his freshman and sophomore year Donny passed his driver's test, allowing for him to drive both himself and a few neighbors to school. This was particularly helpful since the commute to school took about 30 minutes each way. The kids that road with him chipped in for gas.

By the fall of his sophomore year, Donny appeared to be thriving. He was able to obtain a 2.4 grade average which he sustained through the entire year. Despite his success, he grumbled about the dress code, the closed campus, and the strict nature of the classrooms.

Between his sophomore and junior year Donny spent much of his time hopping from one teen party to another, indulging in alcohol and marijuana. For many teenagers this would have simply been a matter of trying adulthood on for size. For Donny, this may well have intensified his depression, as both are known for their depressant effects.

Donny entered his junior year with the expectation of continuing on through all five years at the Academy, a thought that meant for him that he was becoming successful. But as he entered his upper-level classes, he was placed with a mechanics teacher that was known for his high expectations in reading and writing. Donny, still wanting to be perceived as both normal and successful, did not opt for oral exams in this class. The teacher, despite his knowledge of Donny's learning disabilities, did not waver in his expectations and began failing Donny's papers, despite the in-depth knowledge that Donny presented in them. For the first time, it appeared that he might not be able to attend all five years at the academy. Donny's grade point average dropped below a 2.0, and this crushing blow appeared to affected him greatly.

It is at this point in Donny's life that a large number of mounting concerns have been identified and need to be addressed. The following information is intended to serve as a resource for students and practitioners.

In the first section, a sample psycho-educational evaluation and intake evaluation for possible therapeutic treatment can be found. The psycho-educational evaluation is part of the school-based assessment. This is one sample of a report that integrates various measures in order to aid practitioners with interpretation. **The purpose of the intake evaluation for possible therapeutic treatment is to ....**

Sections II through IV provide information about how REBT, Adlerian, and Existential therapies could be utilized to help Donny through this crisis. Information pertaining to each of these therapeutic approaches is provided and sample of how these specific approaches can be utilized in sample sessions.

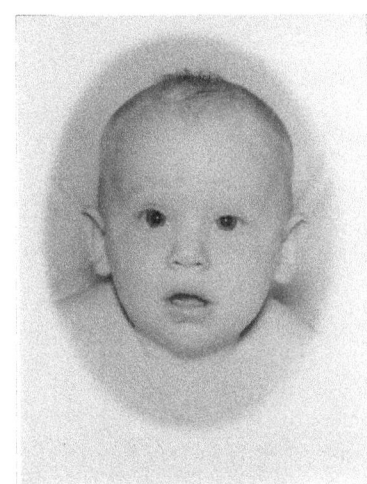
Donny as a baby

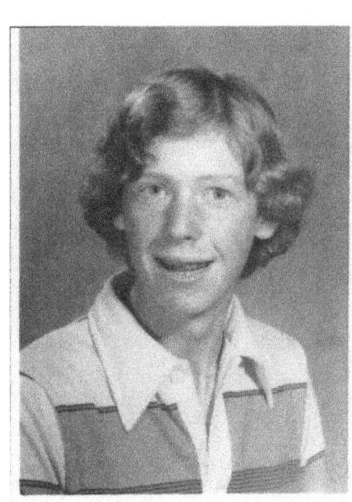
Donny at 17

SECTION I: Evaluation and Intake

Rosemead County Board of Education
Office of Psychological Services
3907 Rosemead Blvd.
Rosemead, CA 91770
626-460-3535
www.rosemead.k12.ca.us

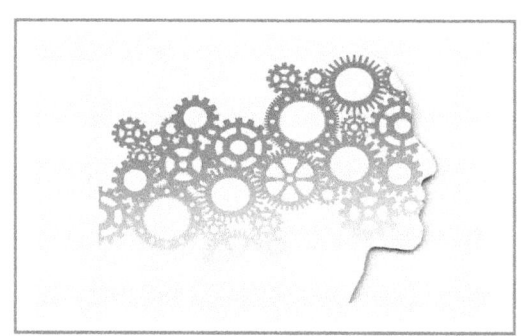

CONFIDENTIAL PSYCHOEDUCATIONAL REPORT

PLEASE NOTE: This is a confidential psychoeducational evaluation report to be kept in a locked file and made available only to those professional school personnel directly concerned with the student. This report MUST NOT BE COPIED OR DUPLICATED WITHOUT PARENTAL CONSENT. If other agencies request a copy, this office will be pleased to supply it directly to them upon receipt of the parent's or guardian's signed release.

Student Name:	Donald "Donny" Kimball	**School:**	Don Bosco Technical Institute
Gender:	Male	**Grade:**	10th
Date of Birth:	5/28/2004	**Age:**	16 years, 9 months
Parents:	Gerald & Lee Kimball	**Examiner:**	Jessica C. Tranquillo, PhD
Home Address:	2101 Rosemead Rd. Rosemead, CA 91770	**Dates of Evaluation:**	3/5/21; 3/8/21; 3/15/21

REASON FOR REFERRAL

Donny is currently a 10th grade student enrolled at Don Bosco Technical Institute. The current Individualized Education Program (IEP) developed in March 2020 includes the classification of Specific Learning Disability (SLD) due to a profile of processing strengths and weaknesses that negatively impact his academic performance. Medically, Donny has diagnoses of Attention Deficit/Hyperactivity Disorder (AD/HD): Combined presentation, depression, dyslexia, migraines, and a seizure disorder. This evaluation was conducted to determine Donny's present level of educational performance. Current measures of Donny's processing abilities, academic skills, and social/emotional/behavioral functioning were requested. The results from this evaluation will be used to guide the decision-making process in developing recommendations and intervention strategies, as may be necessary and appropriate for Donny.

BACKGROUND INFORMATION

All background information in this report was provided by Donny's mother, Mrs. Lee Kimball, and through review of available academic records.

Birth and Developmental History: Donny was the result of a pregnancy in which his mother received routine prenatal care. He was born 10 days late via a lengthy 36-hour delivery. He weighed 7 pounds, 8 ounces at birth. Postnatal history is significant for difficulty being calmed, irritability, an inability to self-sooth, and feeding difficulties. Donny's attainment of early developmental milestones occurred within a timely manner. He babbled and smiled at people by 4 months, sat without support by 9 months, said his first words by 10 months, walked by 12 months, and said two-word sentences by 2 years of age. There were no concerns about his early development or need for any early intervention services.

Medical History: Present from birth, Donny presented with a ptosis of the left eyelid. Concern was noted with the possibility of a tumor behind the eye. An MRI was completed with negative results. However, the same nerve which caused the drooping eyelid also caused partial paralysis of the left side of his face. Surgery was performed to correct the eye lid. By the age of 2, Donny's pediatrician began experimenting with pharmaceutical interventions in an effort to calm his hyperactivity. Donny was initially prescribed Stelazine and Thorazine; however, these drugs appeared to "disinhibit" him. His medication was changed to Ritalin which negatively impacted his sleep. In an effort to find answers to Donny's hyperactivity, a psychologist recommended that Donny be given an electroencephalograph (EEG). The neurologist studied Donny's brain wave pattern and classified it as generalized Grade II dysrythmia – unstable and moderately abnormal. He was subsequently prescribed Dilantin (75mg). His behaviors improved as a result. Additionally, Donny experiences a number of allergies and food sensitivities necessitating dietary restrictions. As a result of dietary changes, noticeable improvement was seen in his eczema. However, his asthma and upper respiratory infections persisted. Donny has diagnoses of Attention Deficit/Hyperactivity Disorder (AD/HD): Combined presentation, depression, dyslexia, migraines, and a seizure disorder.

Family History and Home Behavior: Donny resides with his parents and two younger sisters in Rosemead, California. His parents both graduated from college. His father works as an engineer and his mother is a nurse. There are no family concerns that are impacting or affecting Donny at this time. English is the primary and only language spoken in the home. Family history is significant for depression.

With regards to emotional functioning, Donny presents with a history of mood concerns and behavioral problems. He is currently diagnosed with AD/HD: Combined presentation and depression. His depressed moods are triggered by academic failure and perceived academic inadequacies. Recently, he has made statements about not wanting to live; however, no suicidal attempts or plans were reported. Concern with low self-esteem was endorsed. No medication is taken at this time to address the depression.

Regarding behavior, Donny has a long history of acting out in school. He presents with low frustration tolerance and has limited coping skills to manage his distress (e.g., smokes marijuana on occasion). Deficits related to executive skills (e.g., initiation, problem solving, emotional regulation) were reported for Donny. He struggles to independently manage academic tasks and prefers to wait for an adult to structure or assist with written assignments. He has difficulty following multi-step instructions; which is likely a result of inattention or a lack of effort.

Socially, Donny is motivated to make friends and is described as outgoing and extremely social by his parents. He is often the "center of attention" and can be somewhat "silly" or "disinhibited" at school. He enjoys taking risks and is willing to try things that his friends may be afraid to do (e.g., climbing onto the roof of a house; driving cars fast, etc.). Other kids enjoy hanging around Donny and he is often described as a leader.

During a brief clinical interview, Donny reported that he does not like school and would like to "drop out" and get his GED. However, he expressed concerns with his parent's reaction to his desire to leave high school. He dislikes his shop teacher because he "grades me on writing and spelling; which doesn't make sense because it's shop and I can do all of the mechanical work." He describes his other teachers as "fine." He sometimes gets in trouble at school for "forgetting what he has to do" and "walking out when frustrated." Socially, he has a large group of friends and it is easy for him to make and keep friends. Emotionally, he describes himself as "depressed" because he doesn't like school and he feels like it is getting in the way of him getting a job and being successful. At home, he gets along well with his parents and loves his younger sisters. However, he sometimes feels "dumb" when his younger sister has to help him with his homework. Donny reports having difficulty sleeping as his "mind races" and he "can't seem to shut it off." No eating related concerns were noted. If Donny had three wishes, he would wish "1. To be done with school; 2. To have a good job that I like; 3. To have as much money as I need."

Academic History and Current Academic Performance: A review of records indicates that Donny was first found eligible for special education services in 2nd grade. He attended schools in California and the Greater Boston area including Sycamore Elementary School, El Roble Jr. High, Claremont High School, and Don Bosco Technical Institute. School history is significant for retention in the 6th grade. Review of school records indicates that Donny has been absent 20 days this school year and has received 8 discipline referrals. Discipline referrals include classroom disruption and disrespect.

Academically, Donny presents with a history of reading concerns. During pre-K and kindergarten, he struggled to learn his letters and their associated sounds. In early elementary school, Donny had difficulty with decoding and reading passages. Per parent report, Donny tended to memorize passages once they were read to him, but struggled with completing reading-based tasks on his own. These difficulties continued throughout middle and high school. Writing concerns (e.g., forgetting punctuation, letter reversals) were endorsed; however, he is able to demonstrate generally appropriate math computation skills. Math reasoning is impacted by reading difficulties. With regards to behavior at school, Donny is easily distracted and impulsive (e.g., talking during instruction, running in the halls, calling out answers, etc.). He also demonstrates significant frustration with reading, avoids difficult tasks, and is quick to anger. Donny has been noted to leave class when frustrated. School is reportedly a stressor for Donny and he often attempts to avoid going and skips class on occasion.

Donny is currently in the 10th grade at Don Bosco Technical Institute. The current Individualized Education Program (IEP) developed in March 2020 includes the classification of Specific Learning Disability (SLD) due to a profile of processing strengths and weaknesses that negatively impact his academic performance. According to his current IEP, Donny receives collaborative services in English and math and supportive instruction in science. Donny's first semester grades are as follows: Mechanics (Weatherup) = 20; Algebra 1A (Johnson) = 82; Literature (Harris) = 73; Physical Education (Duncan) = 100; and Biology (Epstein) = 77; and Word History (Grant) = 80.

Donny's mechanics teacher, Mr. Weatherup, completed a teacher information form (2/20/2020) in order to provide information pertaining to Donny's current academic performance. He reports that Donny is a very personable and engaging student who struggles with aspects of reading and writing. With regards to academic skills, Donny does not complete work on time, does not always remember to submit assignments, and struggles with test taking. Regarding academic engagement, Donny often appears bored or not engaged in learning. He asks irrelevant and sometimes inappropriate questions, which can disrupt the learning of other students. Strategies or interventions that benefit Donny in the classroom include extended time, retakes of tests and quizzes, and graphic organizers. Mrs. Harris, Donny's Literature teacher also completed a teacher input form (2/21/2020). She reports that Donny benefits from utilizing speech to text in order to help with written assignments. Socially, Donny has a lot of friends and is "often the center of attention." Other kids are drawn to Donny's charisma and outgoing nature. However, there are times when Donny can be disruptive; which "causes a chain reaction effect. Other students then start to become loud or make inappropriate comments."

Vision and Hearing Screenings

Vision		Hearing	
Date Tested:	2/1/2021	Date Tested:	2/1/2021
Results:	Passed	Results:	Passed

EVALUATIVE PROCEDURES AND TESTS ADMINISTERED
Beery Visual-Motor Integration Test, Sixth Edition (VMI-6)
Behavior Assessment System for Children, Third Edition (BASC-3): Parent, Teacher, & Self-Report Ratings
Behavior Rating Inventory of Executive Functions, Second Edition (BRIEF-2): Parent & Teacher Ratings
Clinical Interview with Student
Consultation with teacher including teacher input forms
Kaufman Test of Educational Achievement, Third Edition (KTEA-3): Selected subtests
Review of Records including: review of pre-referral data and parent input
Test of Auditory Processing Skills, Fourth Edition (TAPS-4)
Wechsler Individual Achievement Test, Fourth Edition (WIAT-4)
Wechsler Intelligence Scale for Children, Fifth Edition (WISC-V)
Woodcock-Johnson IV, Tests of Cognitive Abilities (WJ-IV Cog): Selected subtests

BEHAVIORAL OBSERVATIONS

The following observations occurred within the context of a highly structured one-on-one testing environment with minimal distractions. As such, it is possible that Donnie's behavior will vary in other environments (e.g., a busy classroom).

Donny was a polite, cooperative adolescent who demonstrated variable engagement across tasks. In general, he demonstrated appropriate motivation to complete tasks; however, he benefited from encouragement to persist as tasks became more difficult and on academic tasks. Regarding attention, Donny was easily distracted by outside noises (e.g., people walking around outside the testing room) and had to be prompted back to the task. Test instructions occasionally had to be repeated due to inattention. Donny was verbally impulsive at times (e.g., starting a conversation in the middle of the activity) and was redirected easily with verbal prompts. He would impulsively answer questions and then would immediately self-correct his responses.

During most of the evaluation, Donny displayed an appropriate range of affect; however, when asked to complete challenging tasks, he noticeably appeared frustrated (e.g., sighing, rubbing his face) and asked for breaks. Reading errors were significant primarily for errors of substitution and omission. He struggled with spelling and comprehension, making similar errors in spelling as he did with his reading accuracy. Receptive language was adequate for testing purposes. Expressive language was characterized by fluent speech with good intelligibility. He demonstrated a satisfactory appreciation of paralinguistic features, such as gesture, intonation, and facial expression. Motorically, he ambulated independently with no evidence of balance or coordination difficulties. For fine-motor tasks, he demonstrated an awkward pencil grip resulting in sloppy production of written responses. Given Donny's variable engagement and attention, these results may be an underestimate of his current functioning and should be interpreted with caution. However, despite these concerns, his performance likely reflects his typical day-to-day functioning.

In addition, tests administered on 3/5/2021, 3/8/2021, and 3/15/2021 were conducted with appropriate Personal Protective Equipment (PPE), consistent with our department and district guidelines; which also adheres to CDC recommendations in response to the COVID-19 pandemic. Donnie's performance is not considered to have been negatively affected by the use of these precautions.

TEST RESULTS AND INTERPRETATION

<u>Explanation of standard scores</u>: The results of most psychological tests are reported using standard scores and percentile ranks. Standard scores and percentile ranks describe how a student performs on a test compared to a representative sample group of the same age from the general population. This comparison sample group is called a norm group.

A **standard score** is based on a scale that has an average score (mean) of 100. If a student earns a standard score that is less than 100, then the student is said to perform below the mean, and if the student earns a standard score that is greater than 100, then that student is said to have performed above the mean. There is a wide range of average scores from low average to high average. Most students earn standard scores that fall in the range of 85 to 115. **Scores of <u>85-115</u> are considered to fall within normal limits.**

A **percentile rank** indicates the percentage of children in the norm group who had scores lower than your child's score. A percentile rank does not indicate the percentage of correct answers. For example, a percentile rank of 50 means that 50 percent of children in the norm group had lower scores and 50 percent had higher scores. A percentile rank of 75 means that 75 percent of children in the norm group had scores lower than your child and 25 percent had scores higher than your child.

Standard Score (Mean=100)	T-Score (Mean=50)	Scaled Score (Mean=10)	Percentile Rank	Normative Descriptor Range
>131	>70	>16	98th-99th	Normative Strength
121-130	64-69	15	92nd-97th	16% of the population
116-120	61-63	14	85th-91st	
111-115	57-60	12-13	76th-84th	Normal Limits
90-110	44-56	8-11	25th-75th	68% of the population
85-89	40-43	7	16th-24th	
80-84	37-39	6	9th-15th	Normative Weakness
70-79	30-36	5	3rd-8th	16% of the population
<69	<30	1-4	<2	

Intellectual/Cognitive: An important purpose of the assessment is to provide an estimation of a student's general intellectual ability. Determining cognitive strengths and weaknesses also helps to guide recommendations for the use of specific instructional strategies and intervention techniques, and to evaluate learning potential. The WISC-V was administered and scores are as follows:

Wechsler Intelligence Scale for Children, Fifth Edition (WISC-V)			
Test/Processing Area	Standard Score	Percentile	Classification
Verbal Comprehension Index (Gc)	103	58	Average
Visual Spatial Index (Gv)	119	90	High Average
Fluid Reasoning Index (Gf)	112	79	High Average
Working Memory Index (Gwm)	85	16	Low Average
Processing Speed Index (Gs)	103	58	Average
Full Scale IQ (FSIQ)	106	66	Average
General Ability Index (GAI)	112	79	High Average

General Intelligence: According to the WISC-V results, Donny's General Intellectual Functioning falls solidly within the average range with a Full-Scale IQ score (FSIQ) score of 106; which falls at the 66th percentile. The chances are 95 out of 100 that the FSIQ score is within the range between 100 and 111. It is important to note that the General Ability Index (GAI) was presented as it provides an estimate of general intelligence that is less impacted by working memory and processing speed, relative to the FSIQ. The GAI score of 112 (79th percentile) falls in the high average range.

Cognitive Processing: For the purpose of this evaluation, all basic psychological processes were evaluated which include: Long-Term Retrieval, Short-Term Working Memory, Visual Processing, Fluid Reasoning, Verbal Comprehension, Processing Speed, and Phonological/Auditory Processing. In addition, this examiner also included interpretation of visual-motor ability, orthographic processing, and executive functioning as these areas can impact an individual's achievement as well. For the purposes of this evaluation the WISC-V was the primary measure utilized. Intelligence tests of this nature are often used to identify cognitive strengths and weaknesses as well as to predict a child's ability to learn within the school environment. Tests such as this one, provide an important piece of information regarding an individual's ability to perform measurable tasks requiring various cognitive skills within a controlled testing environment. It is important to note, however, that such tests represent only a portion of what defines intelligence and should be used in conjunction with additional information regarding an individual's capacity to function effectively within his or her environment.

Verbal Comprehension (Gc): Verbal comprehension, or crystallized intelligence, is the breadth and depth of a person's acquired knowledge, the ability to communicate one's knowledge (especially verbally), and the ability to reason using previously learned experiences or procedures. Verbal ability is highly predictive of academic success. There is a strong and consistent relationship to reading, writing, & math throughout school years (e.g., learning vocabulary, answering factual questions, and comprehending oral/written language). Donny earned the following scores on the Verbal Comprehension Index (VCI) of the WISC-V:

Verbal Comprehension/ Gc Subtests	Scaled Score	Abilities Measured/Description
Similarities	11	Verbal reasoning, concept formation. This test requires the child to identify the similarity between two seemingly dissimilar items (words presented orally to the child).
Vocabulary	10	Expressive word knowledge. For the picture items, the child is required to name the pictures in the stimulus book. For the verbal items, the child is required to give definitions for words the examiner reads aloud.

The Verbal Comprehension Index (VCI) measured Donny's ability to access and apply acquired word knowledge. Specifically, this score reflects his ability to verbalize meaningful concepts, think about verbal information, and express himself using words. Overall, Donny's performance on this Index fell in the average range. With regard to individual subtests within the VCI, Similarities required Donny to describe a similarity between two words that represent a common object or concept and Vocabulary required him to name depicted objects and/or define words that were read aloud. He performed comparably across both subtests, suggesting that his abstract reasoning skills and word knowledge are similarly developed at this time.

Visual Spatial (Gv): Visual Processing is the broad ability that allows one to perceive, manipulate, and think with visual patterns and stimuli, and to mentally rotate objects in space; this ability facilitates performance on tasks with visual-spatial stimuli. Moreover, the input has to be synthesized simultaneously, such that the separate stimuli are integrated into a group or conceptualized as a whole. It assesses one's ability to evaluate visual details and understand visual spatial relationships in order to construct geometric designs from a model. This skill requires visual spatial reasoning, integration and synthesis of part-whole relationships, attentiveness to visual detail, and visual-motor integration. Donny earned the following scores on the Visual Spatial Index (VSI) of the WISC-V:

Visual Spatial/ Gv Subtests	Scaled Score	Abilities Measured/Description
Block Design	14	Visual/spatial perception and organization. This test requires the child to view a constructed model or a picture in the stimulus book, and use red-and-white blocks to re-create the design within a specified time limit.
Visual Puzzles	13	Visual/spatial reasoning, mental non-motor construction, visual working memory. Examinee is asked to view a completed puzzle and select three pieces that together would reconstruct the puzzle.

In this area, Donny exhibited performance that fell in the high average range. The VSI is derived from two subtests, Block Design and Visual Puzzles. During the Block Design subtest, Donny viewed a model and/or picture and used two-colored blocks to re-create the design. Visual Puzzles required him to view a completed puzzle and select three response options that together would reconstruct the puzzle. Donny performed comparably across both subtests, suggesting that his visual-spatial reasoning ability is equally developed, whether solving problems that involve a motor response or solving problems with unique stimuli that must be solved mentally and do not involve feedback about accuracy.

Fluid Reasoning (Gf): Fluid reasoning is defined as novel problem solving and reasoning. This type of ability de-emphasizes prior learning. It includes the ability to reason, form concepts through induction and deduction. It often requires the integration of verbal and nonverbal thinking. The ability to reason inductively requires the student to reason from the part to the whole or from the specific to the general. In deductive reasoning activities, the student is given general information and is required to infer a conclusion, implication, or specific example. Donny earned the following scores on the Fluid Reasoning Index (FRI) of the WISC-V:

Fluid Reasoning/ Gf Subtests	Scaled Score	Abilities Measured/Description
Matrix Reasoning	12	Visual problem solving, classification and spatial ability, knowledge of part-whole relationships. Requires the examinee to select the missing piece to complete a pattern.

Figure Weights	12	Quantitative fluid reasoning and induction. On Figure Weights, the child is asked to look at a picture of a scale with a missing weight and identify the weight that would keep the scale balanced.

Overall, Donny's performance on the FRI fell in the high average range. The FRI is derived from two subtests, Matrix Reasoning and Figure Weights. Matrix Reasoning required Donny to view an incomplete matrix or series and select the response option that completed the matrix or series. On Figure Weights, he viewed a scale with a missing weight(s) and identified the response option that would keep the scale balanced. He performed comparably across both subtests, suggesting that his perceptual organization and quantitative reasoning skills are similarly developed at this time.

Working Memory (Gwm): The Working Memory Index (WMI) on the WISC-V requires registering and holding information in immediate awareness briefly and then using that information within a few seconds, before it is forgotten. Success on these tasks requires the ability to retain information temporarily in memory, and in some instances, perform an operation with it. Subtests within this index involve attention, concentration, and auditory and visual discrimination. It also reflects the student's ability to arrange input in sequential order to solve problems, where each idea is linear and related to the preceding one. Attention is a prerequisite condition supporting short term memory. Donny earned the following scores:

Working Memory/ Gwm Subtests	Scaled Score	Abilities Measured/Description
Digit Span	7	Auditory short-term and working memory. The Digit Span Forward task requires the child to repeat numbers in the same order as read aloud by the examiner. Digit Span Backward requires the child to repeat the numbers in the reverse order of that presented by the examiner.
Picture Span	8	Visual working memory and working memory capacity. Picture Span requires the child to memorize pictures and identify them in order on subsequent pages.

Donny's performance on the WMI is slightly low compared with other children his age. Donny experienced the most difficulty on subtests in this area; which is likely related to inattention. There were times when Donny would ask for repetition, even when the instructions indicated that the examiner could not repeat subtest items.

Within the WMI, Picture Span required Donny to memorize one or more pictures presented on a stimulus page and then identify the correct pictures (in sequential order, if possible) from options on a response page. On Digit Span, he listened to sequences of numbers read aloud and recalled them in the same order, reverse order, and ascending order. He performed similarly across these two subtests, suggesting that his visual and auditory working memory are similarly developed or that he verbally mediated the visual information on Picture Span subtest.

Processing Speed (Gs): Cognitive processing speed is a measure of the speed and efficiency in performing automatic or very simple cognitive tasks, particularly when required to maintain focused attention. Processing speed refers to how quickly the person works on easy, routine tasks, such as scanning visual material and making a rapid pencil response. Research suggests that when mental operations are speedy, more information can be processed without overloading the cognitive system. If processing speed is slow the person may have difficulty keeping up with written work. Donny earned the following scores on the Processing Speed Index (PSI) of the WISC-V:

Processing Speed/ Gs Subtests	Scaled Score	Abilities Measured/Description
Coding	10	Graphomotor coordination, short-term memory. It requires the child to copy symbols that are paired with simple geometric shapes or numbers within a specified time limit.
Symbol Search	11	Visual discrimination, decision making speed, psychomotor speed. Child scans a search group and indicates whether the target symbol(s) matches any of the symbols in the search group (timed).

Donny scored within the average range in the area of processing speed. The PSI is derived from two timed subtests, Coding and Symbol Search. Donny demonstrated even performance across subtests within the PSI. On the Coding subtest, she used a key to copy symbols that corresponded with numbers. Conversely, on the Symbol Search subtest, Donny was required to scan a group of symbols and indicate if the target symbol was present. He worked very quickly when scanning rows of symbols to mark the target. His performance suggests that her associative memory, graphomotor speed, and visual scanning ability are evenly developed.

Long-Term Storage & Retrieval (Glr): Long-Term Storage & Retrieval is the broad ability both to store information in long-term memory and to retrieve that information fluently and efficiently. It requires that the student demonstrate focused, sustained, and selective attention, code and store the newly learned information, and integrate auditory and visual stimuli. Also, the student has to generate strategies to facilitate the efficient retrieval of the newly learned paired association from storage. This is not about how much information you can store, but reflects how efficiently you can retrieve the information upon demand. Donny's scores are as follows:

Long-term Retrieval/ Glr Subtests	Standard Score	Abilities Measured/Description
KTEA-3 Object Naming Facility	94	Measures the ability to automatically retrieve the name of objects from his lexical store.
KTEA-3 Associational Fluency	111	Measures the ability to recall information using semantic and phonetic cues.
WJ-IV Cog Story Recall	111	Measures listening ability and reconstructive

			memory.
WJ-IV Cog Visual-Auditory Learning		100	Measures the ability to learn, store, and retrieve a series of visual-auditory associations (rebuses).

Donny was administered subtests from the Kaufman Test of Educational Achievement, Third Edition (KTEA- 3) in order to obtain a measure of long-term retrieval. On the KTEA-3, Donny earned an Oral Fluency Composite score of 103 (58th percentile). While Rapid Automatic Naming (RAN) subtests (e.g., Object Naming Facility) only require minimal memory retrieval skills, the Associational Fluency subtest is a timed measure of word retrieval skills that combines speed of retrieval with memory. A stronger performance on Verbal Fluency (frontal brain regions) versus Rapid Automatic Naming subtest suggests better retrieval speed of language-related tasks, which tends to facilitate passage comprehension skills compared with fluency.

Additional information also obtained in order to provide more information regarding Donny's long-term memory. Donny was administered the Long-Term Retrieval subtests from the Woodcock-Johnson IV Tests of Cognitive Abilities (WJ-IV Cog). On the WJ-IV Cog, he earned a Long-Term Retrieval Composite score of 105 (63rd percentile); which falls solidly within the average range. On the Story Recall subtest, Donny was asked to listen to stories and recall as much of the story as he could remember. The stories increased in length and were not repeated. Donny performed well within the high average range on this task. He was average when asked to learn the word or concept associated with a particular rebus (or drawing) and then read phrases and sentences composed of those drawings.

Phonological/Auditory Processing (Ga): Phonological processing is a form of auditory processing and refers to the use of the sound structure of oral language to "make sense out of" reading, writing, listening, and speaking. Selected subtests from the Test of Auditory Processing Skills, Fourth Edition (TAPS-4) were administered to Donny in order to evaluate his phonological processing skills. Donny scored as follows:

Test of Auditory Processing Skills, Fourth Edition (TAPS-4)		
Auditory Processing/ Ga Subtests	Standard Score / Scaled Score	Abilities Measured/Description
Phonological Processing Index	**72**	**Assesses phonological structure and then using that structure for further language processing.**
Word Discrimination	6	Assesses word discrimination skills.
Phonological Deletion	2	Assesses phonological deletion; a phonemic awareness skill important for the development of reading and spelling.
Phonological Blending	5	Assesses phonological blending; a phonemic awareness skill important for the development of reading and spelling.

Subtests from the Phonological Processing Index provide a quick assessment of abilities that allow individuals to discriminate between sounds within words, segment words into smaller parts (morphemes), and blend letter sounds (phonemes) into words. All these skills are important to reading. Donny performed in the below average range with his phonological processing skills. He struggled with discriminating between sounds in words, deleting syllables and phonemes within words, and synthesizing or blending sounds together to form words.

Possible impact on academic achievement: Phonological processing weaknesses and deficits may affect a student's ability to identify and separate discrete sound "chunks," as well as to synthesize or blend sounds together to form words. This will negatively impact their ability to learn and read "new"/unknown words. Phonological awareness provides students with an important tool for understanding the link between written and spoken language. These problems most directly affect reading and spelling development and are manifested by difficulty segmenting words into parts, recognizing and producing rhymes, blending phonemes to make words and adding, deleting and substituting sounds in words to make new words.

Visual-motor integration is the coordination of visual and motor skills that involve the sensory motor areas (fine and gross-motor tasks). It is the ability to use visual cues (sight) to guide movement. Children with weak visual-motor integration skills typically have trouble copying from the board. They are usually unable to organize, write and draw between lines. To assess his visual-motor processing, Donny completed the VMI-6; which is a paper and pencil measure of visual-motor skill based on one's ability to copy progressively complex, specific geometric designs. Donny performed within the average range with a standard score of 98, 45th percentile.

Orthographic Processing is the visual system one uses to form, store, and recall words. When reading, individuals look at letters and words on the page and use their knowledge of sound/symbol relationships to sound out tricky/unknown words. Over time, the visual memory of this word makes it a solid memory in the brain to be called on later. A word memorized in its entirety is called a sight word. Orthographic processing, or coding, is the skill or ability to use orthographic knowledge to read and spell words. The WIAT-4 was utilized to assess Donny's orthographic processing skills. The subtests that comprise this cluster include Orthographic Fluency and Spelling. Donny scored as follows:

Wechsler Individual Achievement Test, Fourth Edition (WIAT-4)		
Orthographic Processing	Standard Score	Abilities Measured/Description
Orthographic Fluency	72	Measures an examinee's orthographic lexicon or sight vocabulary.
Spelling	69	Written spelling of dictated words.

The subtests involved in this composite involve processing orthographic representations by retrieving them from long-term memory (Spelling) or recognizing / naming them with automaticity (Orthographic Fluency). Therefore, this composite involves both the receptive (reading) and expressive (spelling) components of orthographic processing. Donny's performance yielded an overall Orthographic Processing Composite score of 70, 2nd percentile; which is indicative of very low performance. He struggled with reading irregular words fluently and with his spelling skills.

Executive Functioning: This section contains information about Donny's "executive functioning," which refers to a cluster of self-regulation and mental control abilities. These tasks tap skills such as planning and organization, strategy use, sustaining attention, self-monitoring (keeping track of your own performance), impulse control, mental flexibility, and fluency (performing simple or known skills quickly and smoothly). Ratings were completed via administration of the Behavior Rating Inventory of Executive Function, Second Edition (BRIEF-2). Donny was rated by his mother and his Literature teacher, Mrs. Harris. Scores are as follows:

T-Score	Classification
70+	***Clinically elevated (Many more concerns than are typically reported)
65-69	**Potentially Clinically Elevated (More concerns than are typically reported)
60-64	*Mildly Elevated (Somewhat more concerns than are typically reported)
40-59	Average score (Typical levels of concern)
<40	Low score (Fewer concerns than are typically reported)

Behavior Rating Inventory of Executive Function, Second Edition (BRIEF-2)			
Scales	Behavioral Description	T-Score Parent	T-Score Teacher
Clinical Scales			
Inhibit	Control impulses; appropriately stop own behavior at the proper time	66**	44
Self-Monitor	Keep track of the effect of own behavior on others	60*	43
Shift	Move freely from one situation, activity, or aspect of a problem to another as the situation demands; transition; solve problems flexibly	65**	58
Emotional Control	Modulate emotional responses appropriately	62*	45
Initiate	Begin a task or activity; independently generate ideas	61*	78***
Working Memory	Hold information in mind for the purpose of completing a task; stay with, or stick to an activity	64*	74***
Plan/Organize	Anticipate future events; set goals; develop appropriate steps ahead of time to carry out an associated task or action; carry out tasks in a systematic manner; understand and communicate main ideas or concepts	58	63*
Task-Monitor	Check work; assess performance during or after finishing a task to ensure attainment of goal	61*	68**
Organization of Materials	Keep workspace, play areas, and materials in an orderly manner	60*	62*
Composites			
Behavioral Regulation Index	The BRI represents a child's ability to regulate and monitor behavior effectively. It is composed of the Inhibit and Self-Monitor scales.	65**	44
Emotional Regulation Index	The ERI represents a child's ability to regulate emotional responses, including in response to changing situations. It is composed of the Shift and Emotional Control scales	65**	51
Cognitive Regulation Index	The CRI represents a child's ability to control and manage cognitive processes and problem solve effectively. It is composed of the Initiate, Working Memory, Plan/Organize, Task-Monitor, and Organization of Materials scales	62*	70***
Global Executive Composite	The GEC is an overall summary score that incorporates all of the BRIEF-2 Clinical scales	64*	60*

One or more of the individual BRIEF-2 scales were elevated across raters and settings, suggesting that Donny exhibits difficulty with various facets of executive function. Specific difficulty was identified with aspects of behavioral and emotional regulation (i.e., inhibit, self-monitor, emotional control, and initiate) from the perspective of Donny's mother. At home, Donny struggles to control his impulses, keep track of the effect of his behavior on others, move freely from one situation or activity to another as the situation demands, and modulate his emotional responses appropriately. Conversely, at school, Donny does not experience difficulty with his behavioral or emotional regulation skills from the perspective of his Literature teacher. The Cognitive Regulation Index was identified as problematic across raters and settings. Specifically, Donny was rated as experiencing difficulty with initiating tasks, working memory, task-monitoring, and organization of materials across settings. At school, he also struggles with anticipating future events, setting goals, and developing appropriate steps ahead of time to carry out the task or action. Deficits in the area of executive functioning can negatively impact academic performance.

Academic Functioning: Donny was administered the WIAT-4 which measures academic achievement and consists of a number of subtests that form composite scores. Nationally normed, standardized tests are not aligned with California's CPS (California Performance Standards) standards. Therefore, individually administered achievement tests may vary from an individual's classroom performance in various academic areas. Standardized achievement assessment conducted by this examiner will serve as supplemental information to school data and performance on other group/individual standardized tests; as well as progress monitoring data. Donny earned the following scores:

Wechsler Individual Achievement Test, Fourth Edition (WIAT-4)			
Composite / Subtest	Standard Score 95% C.I.	Percentile	Descriptor
Total Achievement	**63 (58-68)**	**.7**	**Extremely Low**
Reading Composite	79 (72-86)	8	Very Low
Word Reading	81 (75-87)	10	Low Average
Reading Comprehension	81 (68-94)	10	Low Average
(Oral Reading Fluency) *	(73)	(4)	(Very Low)
Mathematics Composite	85 (79-91)	16	Low Average
Math Problem Solving	83 (76-90)	13	Low Average
Numerical Operations	90 (82-98)	25	Average
Written Expression Composite	54 (46-62)	.1	Extremely Low
Spelling	69 (61-77)	2	Extremely Low
Sentence Composition	73 (62-84)	4	Very Low
Essay Composition	40 (26-54)	<.1	Extremely Low

*Subtests in parentheses do not factor into composite scores

Reading: The basic reading subtest, Word Reading, is a measure of sight word vocabulary and decoding that requires the student to read isolated letters and words. Donny's performance is within the low average range for his age. His mistakes were noted to include substitutions of words that were visually similar to the target word. For example, he read "think" for "that." Reading fluency is the ability to read words at an appropriate rate. Donny's overall reading fluency score fell within the very low range. The number of errors made by Donny on the oral reading fluency passages was unusually high and his reading rate was unusually slow when compared to same-aged peers. Reading comprehension is the skill of understanding what one has read. It includes literal and inferential comprehension, vocabulary, and reasoning. Donny's reading comprehension score fell within the low average range. He was able to answer 54% of literal comprehension, 64% of inferential comprehension, 100% of narrative comprehension, and 62% of expository comprehension questions accurately.

Mathematics: Math Calculation evaluates an individual's ability to complete pencil and paper math problems. It involves computation of math problems with increasing level of difficulty involving all basic operations. Donny's performance on the Numerical Operations subtest yielded a score in the average range compared to same age peers. In general, Donny was able to demonstrate knowledge of basic math skills, add and subtract with single-, two-, and three-digit numbers, multiply with multiple digits, and complete problems requiring knowledge of the order of operations, long division, algebra, and geometry. Qualitative behavioral observations suggests difficulty with lining up numbers on computational problems, which led to errors on this task.

The Math Problem Solving subtest assesses the ability to reason mathematically. It tests required skills in analyzing and solving real-life problem situations. To solve such problems, it is necessary to recognize the procedure to be followed, identity relevant data and then perform the required calculation. Donny's score is within the low average range for his age. He was able to order numerals, identify place value, interpret graphs, measure an object, add & subtract objects, interpret a number line, complete problems requiring knowledge of money, and complete single-operation word problems. Conversely, Donny struggled with reading an analogue clock, completing number patterns, ordering fractions, interpreting transformation of figures, finding the perimeter, multi-step problems, and solving probability problems.

Written Language: Written Expression refers to the academic skill of formulating and writing sentences that clearly express ideas and follow the rules of informal standard American English. Donny performed in the very low range with building sentences when provided with a target word and combining sentences. When asked to write an essay when provided with a prompt, he struggled with writing in a manner that expressed his ideas in a complete sentence using appropriate syntax (word order) and semantics (word meanings). He also struggled with the mechanics of writing and would forget to capitalize words or he would utilize incorrect punctuation. Donny's spelling performance fell in the extremely low range when compared with same-aged peers with a number of phonetic errors identified.

Social-Emotional: The Behavior Assessment System for Children – Third Edition (BASC-3) was administered in order to obtain more detailed information regarding Donny's social-emotional and behavioral functioning. The BASC-3 is an assessment tool used to evaluate children and adolescent's behavior as rated by adults who know the child best. The BASC-3 measures numerous aspects of behavior and personality, including positive (adaptive) and negative (clinical) dimensions. In addition to specific scale scores, the BASC-3 generates composite scores that reflect the overall severity of externalizing types of problems, internalizing problems, school problems, and deficits in adaptive behavior. Donny's mother and his classroom teachers, Mr. Weatherup, Ms. Johnson, and Mrs. Harris, served as informants. The following chart is provided as a guide to *T*-score interpretation:

Clinical Scales	Adaptive Scales

70+	Clinically Significant	70+	Very High
60-69	At Risk	60-69	High
41-59	Average	41-59	Average
31-40	Low	31-40	At-Risk
30 and below	Very Low	30 and below	Clinically Significant

Several scales on the BASC-3 measure the validity of the test-taker's responses. The validity scales suggest that all raters responded in a consistent, accurate, and forthcoming manner when describing Donny's behavior. The following are parent and teacher scores for Donny on this test:

Behavior Assessment System for Children, Third Edition (BASC-3)					
Scales	Description	Weatherup T-Score	Harris T-Score	Johnson T-Score	Parent T-Score
Clinical Scales					
Hyperactivity	The tendency to be overly active, rush through work or activities and act without thinking	74**	42	42	54
Aggression	The tendency to act in a hostile manner that is threatening to others	64*	43	46	61*
Conduct Problems	Socially deviant and/or disruptive behaviors that are related to the diagnostic category of Conduct Disorder, including symptoms such as cheating at school, stealing, lying, and disregard for others' rights and feelings	74**	43	43	67*
Anxiety	Feelings of nervousness, worry, and fear; the tendency to be overwhelmed by problems	57	68*	67*	73**
Depression	Feelings of unhappiness, sadness, and dejection; a belief that nothing goes right	60*	70**	48	72**
Somatization	The tendency to be overly sensitive and complain about relatively minor physical problems and discomforts	45	44	44	39
Atypicality	The tendency to behave in ways that are considered "odd" or commonly associated with psychosis	43	47	44	51
Withdrawal	The tendency to evade others and avoid social contact	42	72**	51	51
Attention Problems	The tendency to be easily distracted and unable to concentrate more than momentarily	62*	47	44	51
Learning Problems	The presence of academic difficulties, particularly understanding or completing homework	85**	41	59	
Adaptive Scales					
Adaptability	The ability to adapt to change in the environment	44	44	55	34*
Social Skills	Skills that are necessary for interacting successfully with peers and adults in home, school, and community settings	54	46	58	39*
Leadership	Skills associated with good community and school adaptation	51	49	55	37*
Functional Communication	Ability to express ideas and communicate in ways that others can easily understand	54	51	49	37*
Activities of Daily Living	Ability level relative to various basic self-care skills and everyday tasks, such as completing chores, attending to personal safety, and brushing teeth				48
Study Skills	Skills that are conductive to strong academic performance, including organizational skills and good study habits	35*	53	58	

	Composites				
Externalizing Problems	This composite is characterized by disruptive behavior problems such as aggression, hyperactivity, and delinquency	72**	42	43	61*
Internalizing Problems	This composite includes scales that measure depression, anxiety, and similar difficulties that are not marked by acting out behavior	55	62*	53	63*
School Problems	This composite consists of the attention problems and learning problems scales. It reflects academic difficulties, including problems of motivation, attention, learning, and concentration	75**	44	52	
Behavioral Symptoms Index	A measure of overall problem behavior	59	54	45	58
Adaptive Skills	This composite summarizes prosocial, organizational, study, and other adaptive skills	47	48	55	37*

*=at-risk; **=clinically significant

From the parent perspective, Donny demonstrates clinically significant anxiety and depression, a pattern that occurs in 1.8% of the standardization sample. This profile typically indicates high levels of internal distress such as depressed mood, anxiety, and low self-esteem. Donny also exhibited elevations on the BASC-3 externalizing scales of Aggression and Conduct Problems, a pattern that can co-occur with the internalizing disorders noted. This suggests that Donny is exhibiting significant behavioral difficulties in conjunction with his emotional distress. It may be the case that internal emotional distress is causing Donny to act out, or that negative feedback related to his behavioral issues may be resulting in depressed or anxious moods. Given these concerns, the Emotional Disturbance Qualification (EDQ) scale on the BASC-3 was at-risk for unsatisfactory interpersonal relations and inappropriate feelings. The EDQ scale was clinically significant for unhappiness or depression. This scale serves to help determine if Donny's eligibility for ECS would be best categorized by the category of Emotional/Behavioral Disorder (EBD). Adaptively, Donny was rated as demonstrating age-appropriate daily living skills. Elevated parent concerns were noted in the areas of adaptability, social skills (for example, does not always make positive comments), leadership, and functional communication.

Teacher ratings were completed by Mr. Weatherup (Mechanics), Ms. Johnson (Algebra 1A) and Mrs. Harris (Literature). From the perspective of his teachers, Donny demonstrates anxious and depressed moods to varying degrees in his classes. Consistently noted across raters, Donny he often is irritable, is pessimistic, says, "I can't do anything right," and says, "tests make me nervous." Additionally, withdrawal was very elevated from the perspective of Mrs. Harris. In Literature, Donny isolates himself from others and sometimes avoids other adolescents. Given these concerns, the Emotional Disturbance Qualification scale on the BASC-3 was at-risk for inappropriate behavior / feelings and unhappiness or depression from the perspective of Mrs. Harris but not from the perspective of Mr. Johnson or Mr. Weatherup. Otherwise, Mr. Johnson and Mrs. Harris indicated that there were no significant concerns with hyperactivity, inattention, executive functioning (Harris T-Score = 45; Johnson T-Score = 44), conduct problems, aggression, somatization, learning problems, or adaptive behaviors.

Conversely, from the perspective of Mr. Weatherup, Donny experiences significant behaviors related to hyperactivity, aggression, and conduct problems. Specifically, he argues when denied his own way, almost always defies his teacher, often gets into trouble, uses foul language, and almost always speaks out of turn during class. With regards to inattention, Mr. Weatherup identified a number of behaviors related to Donny's diagnosis of AD/HD including being easily distracted and having difficulty paying attention. These behaviors are having a negative impact on his performance in class.

Donny also completed a <u>Behavior Assessment System for Children, Third Edition</u> (BASC-3) self-report. He completed the measure in a meaningful and cooperative manner.

<u>Behavior Assessment System for Children, Third Edition (BASC-3): Self-Report</u>		
<u>Scales</u>	<u>Description</u>	<u>Self-Report T-Score</u>
Clinical Scales		
Attitude to School	Feelings of alienation, hostility, and dissatisfaction regarding school	82**
Attitude to Teachers	Feelings of resentment and dislike of teachers; beliefs that teachers are unfair, uncaring, or overly demanding	88**
Sensation Seeking	The tendency to take risks and seek excitement	82**
Atypicality	The tendency towards bizarre thoughts or other thoughts and behaviors considered "odd"	43
Locus of Control	The belief that rewards and punishments are controlled by external events and people	61*
Social Stress	Feelings of stress and tension in personal relationships; a feeling of being excluded from social activities	52
Anxiety	Feelings of nervousness, worry, and fear; the tendency to be overwhelmed by problems	41
Depression	Feelings of unhappiness, sadness, and dejection; a belief that nothing goes right	74**
Sense of Inadequacy	Perceptions of being unsuccessful in school, unable to achieve one's goals, and generally inadequate	87**
Somatization	The tendency to be overly sensitive to, to experience, or to complain about relatively minor physical problems or discomforts	42
Attention Problems	The tendency to report being easily distracted and unable to concentrate more than momentarily	62*
Hyperactivity	The tendency to report being overly active, rushing through work or activities, and acting without thinking	58
Adaptive Scales		
Relations with Parents	A positive regard towards parents and a feeling of being esteemed by them	46
Interpersonal Relations	The perception of having good social relationships and friendships with peers	61
Self-Esteem	Feelings of self-esteem, self-respect, and self-acceptance	30**
Self-Reliance	Confidence in one's ability to solve problems; a belief in one's personal dependability and decisiveness	37*
Composites		
School Problems	A broad measure of adaptation to school	95**
Internalizing Problems	A broad index of inwardly directed distress that reflects internalizing problems a child may experience	59
Inattention/Hyperactivity	A composite scale that represents an aggregated score	61*

	containing scales most directly related to ADHD symptomology	
Emotional Symptoms Index	The most global indicator of serious emotional disturbance, particularly internalizing disorders.	68*
Personal Adjustment	A composite containing scales related to relations with parents, interpersonal relations, self-esteem, and self-reliance	42

These results indicate a very negative attitude toward school for Donny, at clinically significant levels. Donny reports that he doesn't like thinking about school but does care about school. He almost always feels that school is boring and that he often feels like he wants to quit school. Donny also displays a negative attitude towards his teachers. Although he feels that some teachers care about him, he does not feel that his teachers understand him and are only sometimes proud of him. He feels like his teacher often gets mad at him for no reason and that sometimes teachers are unfair.

Elevation is also reported in a sense of inadequacy, which generally relates to feelings of inadequacy regarding school. For example, Donny reports that he never quite reaches his goals and that most things are harder for him than for others. He notes that he often quits easily and would rather quit than fail. Donny is almost always disappointed with his grades and often he wants to do better but he can't. Related to this area, Donny's responses also suggest problems with feelings of self-reliance. He reports that if he has a problem, he cannot usually work it out; though he also says that often he can solve difficult problems by himself. When asked, Donny reports that he can't solve academic problems by himself but is able to solve problems related to interpersonal relationships.

Donny also sees himself as having some elevation in attention problems. He reports that people tell him that he should pay more attention and that often he has trouble paying attention to the teacher. He notes that he often forgets to do things and often is easily distracted.

Finally, Donny endorsed BASC-3 items that resulted in a clinically significant Depression scale score; which is consistent with his diagnosis of depression. Specifically, Donny reports that he just doesn't care anymore, nothing ever goes right for him, he almost always feels that life is not worth living, and his life is getting worse and worse. He reports having low self-esteem (specifically when related to academics), and finds things to be outside of his control (i.e., elevated Locus of Control scale score).

On a positive note, Donny reports a good relationship with his parents and friends. Specifically, he gets along well with his parents, his parents are easy to talk to, his parents are often proud of him, he gets along well with others, and kids like to be around him.

SUMMARY AND RECOMMENDATIONS

Donny is currently a 10th grade student enrolled at Don Bosco Technical Institute. The current Individualized Education Program (IEP) developed in March 2020 includes the classification of Specific Learning Disability (SLD) due to a profile of processing strengths and weaknesses that negatively impact his academic performance. Medically, Donny has diagnoses of Attention Deficit/Hyperactivity Disorder (AD/HD): Combined presentation, depression, dyslexia, migraines, and a seizure disorder. The results from this evaluation will be used to guide the decision-making process in developing recommendations and intervention strategies, as may be necessary and appropriate for Donny.

Findings from the current assessment indicate that Donny is an adolescent male of high average intellectual functioning (SS = 112). In general, Donny's broad average performance on tasks of verbal reasoning and on tasks of fluid, non-verbal reasoning suggests that his ability to comprehend and apply information is generally sufficient to allow him to understand and master appropriate grade-level concepts and skills. Assessment of additional areas of cognitive processing indicate a pattern of strengths and weaknesses across a number of domains assessed. Abilities were in the broad average range for visual processing, working memory, long-term storage and retrieval, visual-motor integration, and processing speed. Weaknesses were noted with his phonological processing and orthographic processing abilities; which are key cognitive skills that underlies the development of basic reading skills. These basic reading weaknesses can have a negative impact on Donny's ability to read fluently and comprehend what he reads. When asked to spell single words from dictation, Donny performed in the extremely low range with a number of phonetic errors. His ability to build sentences when provided with a target word and combine sentences was very low. When asked to write an essay when provided with a prompt, Donny struggled with writing in a manner that expressed his ideas in a complete sentence using appropriate syntax (word order) and semantics (word meanings). Math was described as a strength from the perspective of Donny's teacher. On a standardized measure of assessment, he performed in the low average range with math reasoning and average with math computation.

Donny's profile should be considered in the context of his AD/HD diagnosis. Children and adolescents with AD/HD often present with difficulties in a variety of cognitive and emotional abilities. Behavioral inhibition, a primary concern in children with AD/HD, leads to further impairment in a variety of executive functions, including self-regulation and cognitive flexibility. These difficulties can impact academic functioning, behavioral presentation, and emotional, and social functioning.

In addition, Donny's current emotional and mood functioning exceeds what would be expected secondary to his diagnosis of AD/HD. He has a history of depressed moods. His depressed moods appear to be exacerbated by his academic difficulties. As a result of these concerns, Donny reports with thoughts of suicide; however, no suicidal attempts or plans were reported. With regards to cognitive skills, individuals with depressive disorders often present with declines in executive functioning (verbal fluency, inhibition, planning), sustained attention, and verbal memory abilities. Research has linked depression to lower perceived cognitive competence and negative academic self-report. Furthermore, children and adolescents with depression tend to have less positive relationships with their teachers and more behavioral problems within the academic setting (e.g., behavioral refusals, noncompliance, etc.).

In summary, it is the examiner's belief that Donny exhibits a phonological-core deficit, which is a term used to describe problems with the phonological underpinnings of learning to read. This phonological-core deficit typically involves some combination of problems with phonological awareness, rapid automatized naming, phonological short-term/working memory, and/or phonic decoding. It can range from mild to severe and is likely the cause of most word-level reading problems. In general, findings from this evaluation are consistent with his previous diagnosis of dyslexia. Additionally, Donny's social-emotional functioning and significant medical history are impacting his academic performance as well. Given these concerns, Donny's parents may wish to share this information with a medical professional and an outside counselor.

A final decision regarding the appropriateness of special education services is the responsibility of the Individualized Education Program committee. The IEP committee is also responsible for determining the type and extent of service delivery. The committee should give careful consideration to the fact that tests are samples of behavior and should view test scores as estimates. Tests scores do not necessarily reflect permanent, unchanging traits. Tests assess developed abilities and scores are therefore, subject to some fluctuation.

Orthographic Processing: Donny demonstrated weakness with his orthographic processing skills. Interventions related to orthography most commonly relate to improving spelling. For example, have Donny use the Look-Spell-See-Write strategy to highlight the visual image of a word for spelling. Print the word to be learned on a piece of paper or index card for him. Make sure that the word is one that Donny can read easily. Donny then looks at the word while reading it aloud, says each letter, tries to create a mental picture of the word, and writes it three times, each time checking it against the card for accuracy. If he makes an error at any point during the three trials, he goes back to the original study-steps. Another idea would be to use a cloze procedure to practice spelling. Give Donny an index card that has a word at the top and then underneath the word written several times with different letters deleted. Gradually, reduce the number of letters provided in the target word. On the last trial, have Donny turn over the card and write the word entirely from memory. This method can be adapted by omitting specific word parts, such as vowels, consonants, consonant blends, prefixes, suffixes, or the irregular element of the word.

Reading Fluency: Fluency is the goal of this assisted cloze reading intervention. Sessions last 10-15 minutes. The teacher selects a passage at the student's instructional level. The teacher reads aloud from the passage while the student follows along silently and tracks the place in the text with a finger. Intermittently, the teacher pauses and the student is expected to read aloud the next word in passage. Then the teacher continues reading. The process continues until the entire passage has been read. Then the student is directed to read the text aloud while the teacher follows along silently. Whenever the student commits a reading error or hesitates for 3 seconds or longer (whether during the assisted cloze or independent reading phase), the teacher stops the student, points to and says the error word, has the student read the word aloud correctly, has the student read the surrounding phrase that includes the error word, and then continues the current reading activity. Optionally, the teacher may then have the student read the passage again (repeated reading) up to two more times as the teacher continues to silently monitor and correct any errors or hesitations.

Written Expression:
- For first drafts, act as a scribe for Donny to allow him to dictate his ideas.
- Allow use of dictation software when appropriate.
- Allow more time for written tasks including note-taking, copying, and tests.
- Encourage learning keyboarding skills to increase the speed and legibility of written work.
- Reduce copying aspects of work; for example, in math, provide a worksheet with the problems already on it instead of having Jack copy the problems.

- In attempting written expression tasks, teachers may wish to utilize the COPS strategy to help Donny monitor his written expression using the following:
    - **C**apitalization: have you capitalized proper nouns as well as the beginning of each sentence?
    - **O**verall appearance: How does my paper look? Is it neat? Is there proper spacing?
    - **P**unctuation: Do I have proper punctuation at the end of each sentence? Do I use my punctuation to create a mood by using question marks and exclamation points? Did I use commas appropriately?
    - **S**pelling: Have I used a dictionary/word bank for any words I am unsure of? Did I have someone else proof read my work?

Executive Functioning: Given the difficulty noted with Donny's executive functioning skills across raters and settings, the following recommendations are offered:
- When completing complex tasks or projects (e.g., organizing her room, writing a paper), Donny is encouraged to break down large goals into small, more proximal goals.
- When setting goals, make sure that goals are concrete (highly specific). Also, write smaller goals down in sequential order so that once one goal is accomplished, Donny will immediately know what the next step/goal is.
- Donny demonstrated some difficulty with working memory. He will likely benefit from information presented in small segments and shorter learning periods with breaks. New information should be repeated and reviewed regularly and teachers/caregivers should ensure that Donny is paying attention before teaching him new information.
- Changing tasks more frequently can alleviate some of the drain on sustained working memory for Donny, whose focus is likely to fade more quickly than his peers. Changing from one task to the next sooner can help restore his focus for a brief period of time. Tasks can be rotated, such that he might work for 10 minutes on math problems and 10 minutes on reading, and then return to another 10 minutes of math.
- Important skills (e.g., academic / work routine) should be completed in the same order each time, which will help Donny to develop habits/routines. When starting a task or a group of tasks, Donny should start with the easier activity and move to more challenging activities. This approach builds behavioral momentum, which makes tasks easier to complete. Donny should be provided with opportunities to select the order in which he completes activities, when possible. This strategy will provide him with a greater sense of control.

Social-Emotional: Providing Donny with a self-monitoring checklist and positive reinforcement system to address self-regulation will be a helpful tool. In addition, teaching Donny to verbally request to take a break when he needs one can help him to calm down when he is frustrated. By taking a moment to collect himself, do something to distract himself, or relaxing (e.g., deep breathing, taking a walk, talking it out with an adult) Donny can return to a stressful situation without incident. Being able to take a break when he is overwhelmed, angry, or overstimulated allows him to learn relaxation techniques and appropriate ways to handle stressful or uncomfortable situations. It is important to teach Donny the procedure for how and when it is appropriate to take a break. The procedure must be clearly defined and limits on how many breaks he can get will need to be identified. Once Donny is on a break here are some options for activities he can do:

1) Deep Breathing – Breathe in for 4 counts and then out for 4 counts, then repeat as many times as needed. Remember to count at a one second per number pace and slow your breathing to match (e.g., Breathe in for 1 Mississippi, 2 Mississippi, 3 Mississippi, 4 Mississippi and out for 1 Mississippi…)
2) Use a "Calm Down" Object – often when we are upset, squeezing a stress ball or playing with something soothing can help to calm us down. Try it! Calm down objects can be anything from sparkle bottles and stuffed animals to stress balls and playdough.
3) Draw or Color – Drawing can be fun and relaxing. Try using markers, crayons, pencils, or paint to express how you are feeling. Sometimes it is easier to draw our emotions than it is to talk about them.
4) Meditate – Meditating can be really helpful in calming down. Find a comfortable position lying down or sitting in a chair and focus on your breathing. Remember when thoughts other than breathing come into your mind just acknowledge them and bring your mind back to your breathing. Don't judge your thoughts, just let them happen.
5) Progressive Muscle Relaxation – Find a chair or spot on the floor and concentrate on your body. Start with your head and scrunch up your face to tense your muscles for a few seconds then relax away the stress. Move to your arms then your shoulders, and finish with your legs, tensing your muscles and then relaxing before moving on.
6) Visualization – Find a comfy spot on the floor or the chair. Close your eyes and focus on your breathing. Start ton imagine a place that makes you feel calm and relaxed. This could be the beach, the forest, some other place you find comforting (e.g., home, grand mom's house, a park, etc.). Try to imagine all the details (e.g., what it looks like, feels like, and smells like).

It has been a pleasure to work with Donny. If you have any questions about the information in this report or need further assistance, please do not hesitate to contact me at School Psychological Services (tranquillo.jessica@mail.rosemeadboe.org or 626-460-3990 x1238).

Jessica Tranquillo

Jessica C. Tranquillo, Ph.D., NCSP
Nationally Certified School Psychologist
Rosemead County Public Schools

Report Completed and Submitted: 5/28/2021

Intake Evaluation for Possible Therapeutic Treatment

Client: Donald Francis Kimball
Clinician: Joanne Mekolichick, MA
Date of Assessment: 5/20/2021

Client's Reported Desire for Treatment:
Client seeking therapy to deal with feelings of depression, his concerns about school, and his concerns with what his future will look like if he does not complete the five-year High School/Mechanical Licensing Program at Don Bosco Technical Institute.

Physical Description:
Donny is a 16 y/o male, approximately 6' tall, very slender, with red hair and bright blue eyes, who arrived on time for his appointment.

Orientation:
Oriented X3. He was able to give his full name, tell me the day of the week, the date, his grade level in High School, and who the current president of the United States is. He was also able to tell me where he was, how he got to the appointment, and why he was here.

Cognitive Assessment:
Client was able to openly discuss his current issues with this therapist. He could provide a background of diagnosis and treatments received throughout his life, including 4 Psycho-Educational Evaluations done by a School Psychologist. He is clearly aware of his learning disabilities and the frustrations they cause. He has been in both individual and family therapy with a psychiatrist for most of his life, but would like a new perspective on treatment so he asked his parents to schedule this assessment. Client appears cognitively intact.

Emotional History:
Client reports that he often suffers from feelings of deep sadness, as evident during the session by the fact that he did not smile, did not laugh, and he exhibited mild motor retardation not connected to any other diagnosis previously provided. Client also stated that he believes that the world is "hopeless. Change can never be made. People judge others by what they can put on paper, and not by who they are as a person or what their abilities are." Client cited his innate knowledge with all things mechanical, stating that his previous treatment provider had spoken of his abilities as almost savant in nature. However, he is getting poor grades in his mechanical classes at school this year because of his inability to spell and use proper grammar, supporting his belief that his knowledge is judged by what he can write.

Medical History:
Client reports that he suffers debilitating migraines that "put him to bed." He suffers photosensitivity and nausea with his headaches, although he does not throw up. Some migraines have lasted for more than one day. His migraine trigger is unknown.

Client reports a Dx of allergies which were severe in childhood. He has been told that he received allergy shots before the age of one (1). Shots were administered this early because his allergies were causing other medical problems for him, including asthma and eczema. When asked, he stated that he did not believe they were the cause of his migraines.

Client reports a Dx of Asthma which is allergy induced. Client uses rescue inhalers PRN.

Client also reports a Dx of epilepsy, although he does not remember having seizures and does not know what kind they are. He has been told that he had a seizure at about 1 and 3 yrs/o. Then, when he was about 9 years old, an EEG confirmed his Seizure D/O and he was placed on medication.

Client also mentioned being born with a Lazy Eye. As a child he had what he considered an unsuccessful surgery. Although they lifted his lid so that he could see, they over corrected and he cannot completely shut his eye now. This over-correction requires him to take drops to keep his eye moist, but they blur his vision. Client plans on having surgery again this summer to correct this problem.

Client reports that he has a paradoxical effect with medications which has made treatment of his various medical issues more complicated. He cited a time when he went to have his wisdom teeth pulled and the sedative used to put him to sleep actually made him more active. He was unable to have his teeth pulled that day.

Mental Health History:
Client reports a Dx of ADHD and self-reports that he is aware that he is much more active than most of his friends. He does not like to sit still, and this makes it hard for him to pay attention in class. He reports that he sleeps approximately 6 hours a night and feels good on that amount of sleep.

Client reports a Dx of Dyslexia which has created many problems for him in school. He is self reportedly very smart, but when he takes tests, it appears as if he is "stupid." Client feels he is unable to show his intelligence level because it is only evaluated on paper. This has caused conflict with some teachers throughout his educational career.

Client reports many periods of deep sadness in his history, which his psychiatrist has Dxd as Major Depression. He is currently not on medication, nor has he ever been on medication for his depression. Client has no Hx of hospitalization due to his depression. He does report periods of suicidality and feeling hopeless about the future of the world and whether people are actually capable of change. Therapist did a suicidal assessment and client does not appear to be actively suicidal at this time. However, if client continues with therapy this treatment provider will reassess on a regular basis. With client's extensive amount of time in therapy it is unclear if the client knows how to answer the assessment questions in a manner that will prevent hospitalization.

He reports that he is unable to filter information when he enters a room. He gave an example of what it is like for him to have a conversation. "Other people can focus on the conversation. I hear all the conversations in the room, I notice the clock ticking, I register how bright the lights are, I feel the temperature of the room, I notice if the room has paint, wall paper, what it looks like, I count the number of tables and chairs. I can't shut the other things out and just focus on what someone is saying to me." Client also discussed what physical touch is like for him. "I don't like to be touched or hugged. Only my little sister gets to do that."

When asked, client reportedly uses drugs recreationally. He reports mostly using marijuana, although states he has tried "some other stuff too." He does not believe it has an adverse effect on medications he currently takes. Client was educated on possible potentiation of medications when used together in relation to any medications he may currently be using for his various medical Dxs.

Family History:
Mother is a registered nurse. As such her children receive exemplary medical care. Both Donny and his youngest sister see a neurologist at Loma Linda Medical Center, an hour away from their home. He reports that his mother is very successful. She is a "float nurse" at the hospital and is able to work on all floors. She is also often called to start an IV if no one else can start it.

Father is an Electrical Engineer who works on classified contracts for the government pertaining to missiles and other classified work for the military. He has been very successful in his career, entering management in his early 30's.

Client has two younger sisters. The older of his two sisters is two years younger than him. He reports that he is very close to her. They hang out in the same circles and have the same friends. He rarely goes anywhere without her. He can't remember a time when they were not close.

Client also reports being very close to the younger of the two sisters. She is eight years younger than him and shares many of the same medical, educational, and emotional difficulties that he does. She appears to be unaware of how his difficulties affect him and reportedly idealizes him. She hangs out with him whenever she is allowed and often spends time with him when he is working on his cars.

Mother's father is still alive and is a "back woodsman" who knows how to "hunt, drink, throw darts, and have fun at the bar." He is reportedly culturally Catholic Irish and his Irish Culture is evident in the home.

Client's grandmother died when his mother was 18 years old in her first year of nursing school. She reportedly died of Ovarian Cancer. She was reportedly raised with both Jewish and Catholic faith influences.

Both grandparents are reported to have struggled with alcohol from time to time.

Father's father is still alive. He is retired, but worked on machinery during his career. He is reportedly Scottish, but his culture was not predominant in the home. He too, is reported to have some issues with alcohol.

Father's mother is still alive. She is reportedly culturally Italian and devoutly Catholic. She is also said to be adventurous and took the children many adventures when they were younger and living in Boston.

Client reports that he was at one time very close to his mother's father, but that relationship has not been as close in the past few years. He does not report being very close to his other grandparents and states that it is hard to keep in touch while they are so far away. Client lives on West Coast and Grandparents on East Coast.

Donny reports being very close to his parents and sisters. He enjoys hanging out with them on Friday nights when they run around, have tickle fights, chase each other, and generally get out their energy from the week of work and school. They end their evening together listening to a podcast of The Dr. Demento Show. Donny very much enjoys this time with his family and reports them to be a support system for him.

Social History:
Client reports having many friends, as he has attended both the local schools (Sycamore Elementary, El Roble Jr. High, and some classes at Claremont High School), and a private High School (Don Bosco Technical Institute) where he is now. He has friends from many different social groups and enjoys all of them. He reportedly enjoys their reactions to the many different "stunts" he pulls when he is hanging out. He himself reports enjoying the adrenaline rush he gets when he is "acting crazy."

Donny reports several very close friendships that he can discuss a range of topics which includes how he is feeling about politics, changes that are occurring in the world, his tastes in music, or his feelings in general. His close friends are aware of his diagnosis and difficulties in school and he enjoys being able to talk to them about his frustrations. Covid-19 has provided him much to discuss in the political arena. He has been able to keep up with friends by phone.

He reports having many hobbies: rebuilding old cars, riding dirt bikes, building forts in the back yard, target shooting with the guns his grandfather has given to him, and hanging out with family and friends.

Educational History:
Client has reportedly struggled with school all his life. His Dyslexia and ADHD make it hard for him to perform as well as his peers. He reports being unable to keep up with his peers as early as first grade, when they began to spell and read. He also reports that ever since he can remember he has had a hard time sitting still and teachers do not like that. They often punish for such behavior.

He reports that some schools have tried very hard to keep up with his differences. His grade school in Boston allowed him to be released from school early each day. When he returned from Boston his Grade School here in California held him back, but in 6th grade allowed him to take some of his classes at the High School level, recognizing that he would benefit from shop classes.

Client reports having attended Junior High School in Claremont as well, with much difficulty. He reports that it was hard to have friends in both 6th and 7th Grade. He felt that he should not have been held back, but he understands that due to underperformance it was necessary.

He now attends Don Bosco Technical Institute. He reports that it was hard for him to get in. He and his parents had several interviews and assessments before the decision was rendered that he would benefit from the mechanical program at the school. His hope was to follow the 5-year program where he would receive a High School Diploma and finish with a Mechanics License and an Associate's Degree. However, at this time it does not appear that he will be able to earn the 4-year High School Diploma, but will receive a State Completion Certificate. Client reports being very frustrated with this as he feels his Shop Teacher in school is responsible for this year's low GPA. The teacher requires perfect spelling and grammar on all work and does not put enough weight on his actual ability to do the mechanical work. This has left the client wondering what his future really looks like.

Work History:
Client is currently employed at a local gas station. He pumps gas and, when time allows, he works on cars on a limited basis. He is being mentored by the owner of the gas station who continually tells Donny how good he is at the mechanical work he is being allowed to do in the shop.

V Axis Dx

Axis I: Major Depression w/o Psychotic Features, ADHD, Dyslexia

Axis II: No PD Dx at this time. No MR Dx.

Axis III: Migraine Headaches, Seizure D/O, Paradoxical Medication Reactions

Axis IV: Educational difficulties due to client's dyslexia which has also led to conflict with some teachers. Possible self-esteem issues due to poor academic performance.

Axis V: 55

Recommendation for Treatment:

It is this clinician's opinion that Donald would benefit from further treatment to include 1:1 therapy to address his issues with school, his depression, and to create a plan for how to deal with moving forward if he does not complete the five-year program at Don Bosco Technical Institute.

Client may benefit in the future from family therapy since it has been utilized in the past. However, at this time his issues are personal in nature and deal with becoming independent with or without a High School Diploma. Therefore, it is important that he deal with these issues in individual therapy first.

This clinician also recommends a medication evaluation with a psychiatrist as client reports that he has had suicidal ideations in the past. He may benefit from the support of an antidepressant in order to reduce some Sxs of depression. He may also benefit from medication to treat his Sxs of ADHD. Since client feels that his ADHD interferes with his ability to fully engage in school, a reduction of Sxs might provide support for some improvement.

It is also this clinician's opinion that Donald would benefit from a Neuropsychological evaluation since he suffers from a seizure d/o, ongoing migraines, ADHD, and Depression. Such an evaluation might be able to provide insight into specific coping skills to help him with school at this time. It might also help to determine if Donald is capable of completing the program at Don Bosco Technical Institute. This information would be beneficial to this clinician and to the client as we move forward with determining what his future will look like.

Finally, this clinician would recommend an updated evaluation with a neurologist to include a current EEG to determine how much his seizure d/o and migraines might be affecting his school work and impacting his depression. This clinician would also recommend a thyroid panel be done through his Primary Care Physician to determine if there is any interaction with his Dx of ADHD.

SECTION II: Rational Emotive Behavior Therapy (REBT)

History of the Founder

Albert Ellis was born in Pittsburgh, PA, in 1913 and then moved to New York City at the age of 4. As a child he was very sick and was hospitalized five times for nephritis and often experienced headaches. Despite his childhood illnesses, he was a bright student who enjoyed writing, philosophy, music, literature, and politics (Capuzzi & Gross, 2007).

Anxious about dating, Ellis became interested in sexual and romantic relationships. With little success with the opposite gender, Ellis challenged himself to talk to 100 women at the Bronx Botanical Gardens (Ellis, 2004). Although he never found anyone to date, he recognized the accomplishment of following through on his challenge and desensitized himself, per self-report, to the fear of rejection.

At the age of 21 he received a Degree in Business Administration from the City University of New York. He began his business career during the Depression by matching pants to suit jackets that were still wearable. He went on to become a personnel manager in a gift and novelty firm. In his spare time Ellis began to write books with little success publishing fiction. When his fiction career did not take off, he began writing about sexual adjustment. Because of his research people began to regard him as an expert and started to ask him questions on the subject. As he began to answer them, he realized that he liked counseling almost more than writing so he applied to and attended The Teachers College at Columbia University from 1942 to 1947. He graduated with his Doctorate in Clinical Psychology (Thompson & Rudolph, 1999; Corey, 1996).

In the early part of his professional career Ellis worked as a therapist in state institutions in New Jersey where they employed Psychoanalytic Methods. As he believed this to be the deepest form of therapy he was analyzed and supervised by a training analyst of the Karen Horney School. From 1947 to 1953 he utilized classical analysis in his professional career. He eventually concluded that psychotherapy was superficial and unscientific so he began to experiment with several other theoretical orientations. Influenced by Adler, Horney, and Fromm he began to question the effectiveness of psychoanalysis.

Between 1953 and 1955 Ellis dove back into philosophy and did a complete review of the major therapeutic techniques being used at the time. By the end of 1954 he was developing a new therapeutic approach. Originally called Rational Therapy (RT), it grew into Rational Emotive Therapy (RET). As Ellis continued to develop his theory, combining humanistic, philosophical, and behavioral therapy it evolved into its current name of Rational Emotive Behavioral Therapy (REBT). Ellis particularly liked the work of Alfred Adler who recognized Stimulus, Organism, Response Theory (SOR) of human disturbance. SOR contended that no experience is a success or failure, but that our perspective of the stimulus helps us to make out of it what suits our purposes. Another main influence on Ellis's theory was Paul DuBois who utilized persuasive forms of psychotherapy to help improve disturbed individuals. Ellis also liked the idea of providing clients with homework to improve their success between sessions, originally utilized by Alexander Herzberg. In 1957 Ellis published his first book on REBT called "How to Live with a Neurotic." Two years later he developed the Institute for Rational Living, designed for therapists to learn how to use REBT in their practice. He utilized workshops as his main mode of education. Then in 1960 he published his first successful book called "The Art and Science of Love." He opened the Albert Ellis Institute to train other therapists in REBT. He continued to see clients, run workshops, and publish books on the various uses of his approach to therapy until his death in July 2017.

Construct of Personality

REBT therapists believe that we have a biological temperament that we are born with, and that our personality is greatly impacted by our parents' morals, values, and the experiences that they have provided to us during our formative years. As we grow, we are also influenced by the social groups we choose to participate in. We continue to carry these influences into adulthood. Humans believe it is important to be accepted and approved of by others. Therefore, emotional disturbances can potentially occur when we care too much about what others think (Wedding & Corsini, 2019).

Biology and Personality

REBT therapists recognize the impact of biology on our personality. As infants we are born with a certain amount of demandingness; reacting to our own needs. Then when we gain language, we begin to sustain emotion based on what we tell ourselves internally. If our tendency is to be negative in our self-talk and irrational in our thinking process, then we will sustain negative emotions. We can, however, with the help of an REBT Therapist, teach ourselves to sustain more positive emotions by applying rational thinking.

Social Influences and Personality

As mentioned above, humans are also nurtured in social groups. Therefore, these groups have an impact on how needy we become as adults. We tend to desire acceptance and try to live up to others expectation. We often define ourselves as "good" or "bad" based on outside approval. This desire to fit in and impress others often leads to irrational thinking.

Social relationships are not bad as long as we do not base our happiness on them. For most people, healthy social and intimate relationships correlate with increased personal efficacy. It is only when we base our happiness on other's beliefs of us, that we begin to see emotional disturbance.

Psychological Influences on Personality

In our day-to-day life, activating events occur that lead to a reaction. It is not the event that causes the reaction, but what we think about the event that creates how we emotionally respond to the situation.

Should, must, and ought, form the basis of most emotional disturbance. They lead us to irrational beliefs about current situations.

There are 4 irrational beliefs that tend to occur in our thought process that cause us to react poorly (Corsini & Wedding, 2005).

1. I cannot stand this noxious event.
2. This event is awful and should not exist.
3. People infer almost "godly power" onto themselves believing that they should hold greater power over the fact that the problem does exist.
4. Because people are unable to change the circumstance with this "godly power" they believe they are a failure to the degree of feeling worthless

Once someone has interjected an irrational belief between the activating event and the unhealthy emotional reaction, they tend to create an irrational thought about how they reacted. This becomes the new activating event. The person now creates a new irrational statement to tell them self, and often have yet another unhealthy emotional reaction to this new irrational belief. People often get so stuck on reacting to their reactions, that their disturbances barely relate to the original activating event.

Human Thinking from an REBT Perspective

REBT Therapists believe that human beings tend toward irrational and negative thinking. Such thinking has self-preservation tendencies. Irrational Beliefs (IB) are rigid, dogmatic, unhealthy, maladaptive, and get in the way of our efforts to achieve our goals in life. They usually consist of demands, musts, and should. Rational Beliefs (RB) are healthy, productive, adaptive, and consistent with social reality (Ellis & MacLaren 2005). Therefore, "Human feelings largely stem from thinking" (Ellis & Harper, 1997).

REBT recognizes that when an experience happens, four basic processes occur at the same time. "1) You perceive or sense: see, taste, smell, feel, or hear; 2) You feel or have an emotion about the situation; 3) You move or act: and; 4) You reason or think (Ellis & Harper, 1997)." For example, you smell chocolate chip cookies baking and you feel happy because it reminds you of your childhood. Then you act on the experience. For instance, you walk over to the newly baked cookies and eat one. Then you have a feeling about the experience, such as happiness. Finally, you create a belief about the experience. If, when you were a child, your mother smiled at you when you grabbed the cookie, then your belief may be "my mother loves me." If, however, you mother slapped you on the hand and yelled at you for eating the cookie, then you may have created an Irrational Belief such as "I am a bad person for wanting a cookie." A therapist can only interrupt this process of irrational thinking in one place. They can help you identify the Irrational Belief you created from the experience. By doing this they can then help you review the experience and find the rational thought.

REBT is a rational therapeutic approach that is based on the idea that we can change our perspective by using rational thinking. This approach postulates that most irrational thinking can be summarized as such: Human beings often believe that wants are actually needs, and that they appear to have the need to condemn themselves, others, and the world, if they do not quickly get what they "think" they need. Consequently, this expectation causes them disturbance cognitively, emotionally, and behaviorally (Ellis & MacLaren 2005). Because cognition is something that we as therapists can access, REBT approaches the emotional disturbance at a cognitive level. By changing the cognition, we see long-term philosophical changes on behavior and emotion.

Through research, Ellis recognized three main core beliefs which are frequently identified in the thought processes of emotionally troubled individuals (Ellis & MacLaren 2005, p. 32-33). These three Irrational Beliefs are the basis of disturbed thinking. They are as follows:

1. "I absolutely must, under all conditions, do important tasks well and be approved by significant others or else I am an inadequate and unlovable person."
2. "Other people absolutely must, under all conditions, treat me fairly and justly or else they are rotten, damnable persons!"
3. "Conditions under which I live absolutely must always be the way I want them to be, give me almost immediate gratification, and not require me to work too hard to change or improve them; or else it is awful, I can't stand them, and it is impossible for me to be happy at all!"

However, in more recent literature, people have expanded the list of Irrational Belief's to make it more comprehensive and easier to understand and utilize during therapeutic sessions. The Irrational Belief's identified are (Corsini, R & Wedding, 2005; Jones, 1969):

1. We must be loved/liked by all those around us.
2. Certain people are inherently evil and people who perform such acts should be punished for those deeds.
3. When things don't go our way, it is horrible.
4. Human misery is externally caused or created.
5. If something is dangerous or causes us fear by obsessing over it, we should keep it from occurring.
6. It is easier to avoid difficulties than to face them.
7. We need someone stronger to rely on.
8. We should be thoroughly competent or perfect in all aspects of our lives.
9. Our past history determines our future behavior.
10. If we have control over everything, then nothing will go wrong.
11. We have virtually no control over our emotions.
12. There is a perfect and correct solution to every situation.

Once a therapist and client discover a Core Irrational Belief, they can begin looking for variations in thought processes (Ellis & MacLaren 2005). Some of the maladaptive processes include:

Awfulizing. This is the tendency to put too much emphasize on a situation. Instead of recognizing that it would be nice if a situation were not as it is, a person tells himself that it is horrible, awful, and the worst thing ever. He proceeds to create a negative idea about himself because of it. For example, a student fails one test. It may or may not impact his grade, but the student falls apart because he does not normally fail tests. Instead of learning from the experience and moving on, he focuses on this one test score and tells himself that he is a failure because of this one grade. By creating this unhealthy thought pattern, he has awfulized this situation. The healthier response, as mentioned above, is to learn from the experience, study longer for the next test, and take better notes in class and move on.

Overgeneralizing happens when a person takes one bad situation and then views it as something that will happen in every circumstance. For instance, if a child goes on a play date and the play date does not go well, that child may then overgeneralize and believe that all play dates will not go well. The child fails to recognize that the friend was having a bad day, and the next play date will likely go better. The child has overgeneralized one experience into future play dates.

Personalizing is when people assume that the world revolves around them. Because of this, they believe that everyone else's actions are due to them as a person. For example, a high school friend fails a test. When he sees you at lunch, he yells at you. Instead of asking if the friend is having a bad day, which would be the healthy response, you falsely assume that he is yelling at you because he does not like you.

Perfectionism. This is the need to do and have everything perfect. For example, a young woman might throw a party for her friend's birthday. When her project does not look like the one on Pinterest, she believes that not only is the party a failure, but so is she. Instead, a healthier response would be for her to recognize that her project looks good even though it does not look like the example.

Other maladaptive thought processes include: jumping to conclusions, focusing on the negative, disqualifying the positive, and minimizing the good things.

REBT therapy sessions differ from other theoretical backgrounds in several ways. First, sessions are often shorter because REBT Therapy is a solution focused approach. Therapists do not allow the client to self-indulge by listening to the client's history or long tales of woe. Instead, they focus on one issue to determine the Irrational Belief that is creating their disturbed emotion. Because of this, sessions are often 30 to 45 minutes long, instead of the more common 50 to 60 minutes.

REBT Therapists do not feel it is necessary to spend several sessions building rapport so that the client has warm feelings toward the therapist. Therapy sessions are limited to working on problem identification and goal setting. In the first session, therapists help clients to identify what they are doing to create distress in life. As a result, clients typically leave the initial session hopeful that they will be able to enact change since there is an understanding of the issues. In turn, the therapeutic relationship is often enhanced. Therapists don't hold themselves above the client and instead function more as teachers. Homework, self-disclosure, and the disputation processes are involved in helping the client to develop the ability to change irrational beliefs to rational beliefs. Humor is a popular technique utilized by REBT therapists. Ellis himself utilizes humor to combat exaggerated thinking (Corey, 1996) and counterattack the over-serious side of individuals. This is a relatively brief therapy in comparison to other therapeutic approaches such as psychoanalysis and existential therapy.

REBT Therapists often employ a rapid-fire technique in order to get to the root of the Irrational Belief. They quickly identify the clients dysfunctional thinking. As they challenge the client to defend their belief the illogical thinking becomes apparent. In light of the client's inability to defend their thinking the therapist begins to dispute the Irrational Belief. They help the client understand why the belief system does not work and how it will lead to further disturbance. Finally, they help the client identify more rational thinking.

People are born with the ability to think rationally and irrationally. Developing a rational therapy of life is a major construct of REBT. There are basic concepts to this therapeutic approach that need to be conceptualized and internalized as the therapist, as mentioned by Corsini & Wedding (2005):

1. The way that people think is influenced by their culture and family group. This influence is greatest during the early years of development. This often elicits irrational thinking.
2. People think, feel, emote, and behave simultaneously. Prior experiences weigh heavily into thoughts and actions.
3. REBT requires a client to engage in and do homework outside of the session. Subsequently less sessions are often required when compared to other therapeutic approaches.
4. To discourage dependence, it is believed that a warm relationship is not a necessary condition of the therapeutic dynamic. It is more important that the client engages in the therapeutic exercises during the session and completes homework assignments for the purpose of unconditionally accepting themselves.
5. REBT is not oriented towards symptom removal, but is oriented towards changing the thinking processes. There are 2 forms of REBT: general (teaches rational and healthy behaviors) and preferential (teaches how to dispute irrational ideas and unhealthy behaviors).
6. Neurotic beliefs come from illogical, self-defeated thinking. Individuals underreact and overreact to situations due to irrational unexamined beliefs.
7. REBT requires a client to accept responsibility for their self-defeating thoughts. Only hard work and practice will correct irrational beliefs and keep them corrected.

By understanding these tenants, this allows therapists to understand and work with clients using this approach.

The therapist guides the client in identifying values that need to be promoted. Capuzzi & Gross (2007; noted by DiGiuseppe, 1999) described the following values:

- self-acceptance (the ability to accept both good and bad about oneself)
- risk taking (the willingness to step out of your comfort zone to achieve a certain goal)
- non-utopian thinking (a lack of expectation that everything around you will be perfect)
- high frustration tolerance
- self-responsibility for disturbance (accepting that your actions created your own emotional state)
- self-interest (identifying one's own interest but not in exclusion to the point of egocentricity)
- social interest (engaging in your community)
- self-direction

- tolerance
- flexibility (the ability to change perspectives based on new information)
- acceptance of uncertainty
- commitment (a willingness to give your time and energy to something that you believe in, or a promise to do something).

In order to help the client identify the irrational beliefs in a therapy session and challenge such beliefs, the ABC Model is used. The ABC Model was developed by Ellis and contends that there is an Activating Event (A), a Belief about the action (B), and a Consequence to the action (C), very often our behavioral response. Activating events do not in themselves cause an emotional or behavioral response. Instead, it is the belief about the activating event that causes the emotional or behavioral consequence. Once the consequences and Irrational Belief are identified, the next step is disputation (D). This process helps the client understand the validity, or lack thereof, of their belief system.

Most of us live by a set of convictions about the world which strongly influence our reactions. We rarely question these ideals even though they may be impractical, unrealistic, and illogical (Ellis & MacLaren, 2005). Therefore, disputation is the primary mode to assess whether a thought process is helpful or harmful to a client's belief system. By challenging rigid and inflexible thoughts, the client will eventually replace them with rational alternatives (Capuzzi & Gross, 2007). Two approaches to help challenge beliefs are used: didactic and Socratic.

The didactic approach is the educational and informational portion of therapy. It defines what Rational Emotive Behavior Therapy is, helps the client understand the difference between rational and irrational thinking, and defines the different faulty thought processes. By educating the client we are setting the stage for Socratic disputation.

The Socratic approach provides questions to the client to allow them to explore their own thoughts, assumptions, and ideas in order to get them to disrupt illogical thinking. Client involvement is key during this portion of the therapeutic process with the goal that they will learn to do this for themselves. When using the Socratic approach four types of disputes are utilized: functional, empirical, logical, and philosophical.

In a functional dispute the therapist is trying get the client to understand how his/her beliefs are affecting behavior in a practical manner. The idea is to determine if the thought process is helping or hindering the belief system. If your thought process is that your teacher hates you and every time your teacher provides you constructive criticism you walk out of the room, how is this effecting your life? The therapist may ask "how is this impacting your ability to succeed in high school?"

The empirical dispute is factual in nature and requires evidence to support the thought processes. It checks whether or not the belief system is consistent with social norms. Questions are often statistical in nature and the therapist requires proof of the belief. For instance, if you believe that you are stupid because you failed an exam, what is the evidence that failing an exam automatically makes you stupid. How many exams have you passed before failing this exam? Why does this specific exam define your intelligence?

Logical disputes help clients identify their own illogical beliefs. It explores how the client has made the emotional leap from desires, to needs, shoulds, or oughts. It challenges a client's idea that something must happen a certain way or things are awful. For example, a therapist might ask: Why is it that you think when your mother yells at you she doesn't love you anymore? It is more logical to help the client come to the conclusion that when his/her mother yells that she is angry not that she does not love them.

The final approach is Philosophical disputation. It helps clients to determine where they derive meaning or satisfaction. When a client's perspective has been skewed by a current problem it leads them to define satisfaction by only one area of their life. This belief is often supported by familial or cultural norms. For example, if you grow up in a town where everyone gets married right out of high school and you want to go to college you may develop an irrational belief that you'll never end up married with kids because you spent four years on your college education. It is more logical to help the client come to the conclusion that with a college education they can better support a family once they get married.

Following (D) a client arrives at an effective new belief or philosophy (E). By creating this new belief system, the client arrives at new and healthy feelings (F). The client is then able to respond to their environment in a more healthy and proactive way. Thus, instead of becoming depressed that a romantic relationship did not work out, blaming oneself for the full demise of the relationship, the client could reach a rational conclusion: "because the relationship did not work out, that isn't the end of the world and I am not a failure. It is foolish to blame myself and I am not wholly responsible for the demise of the relationship." The ultimate effect is minimizing the depressed feelings. While it is ok to feel sad about the ending of a relationship, depression is an unhealthy reaction.

A basic tenet of REBT is that individuals have a belief system that impacts the response to a situation. Initially Ellis called this the A-B-C approach. A stands for the activating event or the antecedent. B stands for the belief system. C is the consequence of the event, which can be positive or negative.

If you look at Donny as an example, he consistently had issues with his teachers. In one potential scenario an activating event might be that Donny got a bad grade on a test. Because he had a learning disability, he believed that everyone thought he was stupid. His most common response was to be angry with the teacher; which created tension within the classroom.

Homework
Homework is an integral part of REBT. It is utilized to teach and help clients generalize what is learned during sessions to everyday life. It helps clients to experiment with various new ways of thinking. Some homework is active, such as when Ellis challenged himself to speak to 100 women. Other homework is introspective and requires the client to complete worksheets or writing activities to understand their thought processes and how to change them. See Appendix A for useable tools.

Example of Therapeutic Sessions
Following is an example of how to use the A-B-C Model of REBT Therapy approach with

Donny, the 17-year-old male described in the first section of this book.

As we move forward in this section, the therapist will be identified with a 'T' and Donny, the client, will be identified by a 'D.'

Based on the intake information provided in Section 1, Donny is suffering from Major Depression. REBT therapy is an effective approach to dealing with clients who are depressed because the focus is not on correcting distorted negative inferences but on addressing irrational beliefs (Capuzzi & Gross, 2007). It is also helpful that the therapist does not permit the client to spend too much time self-indulging on the past, instead guiding them to identify solutions.

Before starting the initial session, it is important to address the limits of confidentiality with the client including harm to self, harm to other, or abuse/neglect of a minor or elder.

Describe to Client What a Session Looks Like

The first thing that must be done in every session is to go over basic paperwork, which includes limits of confidentiality. This must be done before you get to know the person, regardless of what theoretical type of therapy you choose to practice. Find examples of paperwork, and how to have this discussion in the appendix.

Session 1: The first session will focus on identifying a problem and an Irrational Belief (IB). In order to help the client, identify the IB, the ABC Model is employed during the session. The therapist will begin with an introduction, not spending time building rapport, but instead focusing on the issue presented.

Introduction
T – Hi Donny, my name is Sarah. I understand that you have done Psychoanalysis before. Is this true?

DK – Yes

T – Did you like this form of therapy?

DK – No

T – Why not?

DK – All we do is talk. We never get anywhere.

T – I am hopeful that you will like REBT Therapy then. It is very different from Psychoanalysis. We are not going to focus on your past. We are going to talk about current problems and help you find solutions to them. REBT believes that Irrational Thinking is at the root of most disturbance. We are going to find out where your Irrational Beliefs (IB) are and help you learn to develop more rational ways of looking at occurrences in your life. Are you open to giving this new therapy a try?

> *Analysis*: Therapist briefly introduces REBT to the client so there is an understanding of what to expect. This didactic approach is the educational and informational portion of therapy.

DK - Sure

T – So tell me what brought you in to therapy today.

DK– My parents brought me here.

T – Why do you think your parents brought you in?

DK – Because I'm depressed.

T – Do you know what depression is?

DK – Yes. I've been living with it my whole life.

T – Are you depressed?

DK – Yes.

T – Do you have any idea why you are depressed?

> *Analysis:* REBT therapists get to the point quickly in the session and develop a hypothesis about the client. Then the client is given many opportunities to challenge, resist, or bring up evidence to the contrary if the client does not accept the therapist's hypothesis.

DK – School sucks. My shop teacher hates me. He thinks I'm stupid.

> *Analysis*: Here Donny believes that his wants are actually needs, and that his shop teacher needs to like him. Because his shop teacher does not like him, Donny is moving towards condemning others. This is causing his disturbance cognitively, emotionally, and behaviorally. If Donny can learn to change his cognition, we will see long term changes on his behavior and emotions.

T – Why do you think that he hates you?

DK – Because he doesn't care if I understand mechanics. He only cares if I am good at English and Spelling. It doesn't matter that I can do everything that he wants me to do in shop class. It only matters if I spell it right in my journal. He knows that I have learning disabilities and he won't cut me a break. He just keeps giving me F's on my papers and I am going to fail the class.

> *Analysis:* This would be considered the A, or Activating event, because Donny identified

the antecedent to the IB. Donny is also exhibiting the IB that "other people absolutely must, under all conditions, treat me fairly and justly or else they are rotten, damnable persons!"

T – So what do you do when you get the F.

DK – I get angry and leave class.

Analysis: This would be considered the C or Consequence because Donny walks out of class. At this point, Donny does not understand that his IB is leading to the Consequence (C). He believes that the activating event has caused the consequence. He does not understand that his irrational belief is driving his behavior. In this instance his primary irrational belief is: this even is awful and should not exist.

T – And is that effective for you?

DK – No, then I get detention.

Analysis: Most clients are assuming that the detention is the consequence. They do not understand that it is an outcome of walking out of class.

T – So, let's back up for a minute. Let's assume that your thoughts cause your own disturbances. When you get a bad grade, what thoughts go through your head?

DK – I hate him.

T – But what do you think about yourself when you see the bad grade?

DK – Oh great, someone else thinks I'm stupid.

Analysis: This would be considered the B or Belief because Donny has just stated that his teacher thinks he is stupid. The IB identified is that human misery is externally caused or created.

T – Okay, so let's suppose he thinks you're stupid. Why would that be so awful?

Analysis: Donny is demonstrating the maladaptive thought process of awfulizing. He is awfulizing the idea that it is horrible if everyone thinks he is stupid.

DK - Because I'm not!

T – Why should he think your smart? It would be nice if he thought you were smart. It certainly would make your class easier. But why should he think you are smart?

DK – Why shouldn't he? I can probably dance circles around him under the hood of a car. I get all the mechanical work done correctly. I've been working on cars since I was in middle school. I have rebuilt several already.

T – We are not concerned here with what you can do, but with the should. You are a smart kid. Think about this. Why should your shop teacher think you are smart? It is the word 'should' that is bothering you and causing you distress. Can we agree on this for now?

DK - [Silence] Sure.

T – Let's think about this a little more. Where did your "should" come from?

> *Analysis*: This would be considered the D or Disputation, which is an active process that will help Donny assess the helpfulness of his belief system. The type of disputation being utilized here is a logical dispute. A logical dispute helps the client challenge the idea that things 'must' happen a certain way.

DK – It's just what I think. Anyone who talks to me knows I'm smart. Why should I have to prove it on paper. Laughs. Well, there is that should again.

T – But why do you think that? Suppose I think you are the stupidest person I have ever met. Why does that matter? [Silence] Here is what I mean. There is a rational line of thinking here. "I'm smart." But there is also an Irrational Belief. "Everyone else should think so too." Why does the world need to agree with that statement? There are plenty of people who wouldn't care. You seem to think that other people are causing your misery. Why?

DK – Because they are keeping me from going to college!

T – Why do you need to go to college?

DK – So that I can be independent and run my own life.

T – Why do you need to go to college to do that?

DK – So I can be a professional.

> *Analysis*: The therapist is employing a rapid-fire technique in order to get to the root of the IB quickly. This helps the therapist identify the clients irrational thinking.

T – OK, I understand your concerns. They are still based on the word should. There are certainly professionals who did not go to college. We can explore this more in our next session. For now, we need to work on how the word should is affecting how you perceive a situation. I'd like you to do some homework between now and our next session. I am going to hand you this worksheet. Don't roll your eyes at me. I know you have learning disabilities. You can have someone read it out loud to you. If you want, you can write your answers down, or say them into a tape recorder. Whatever helps you identify the answers to these questions. We will talk about them in our next session (See Homework Sheet "Identifying Should, Must, and Need Thinking in Appendix A)

Analysis: Homework is provided at the end of the session in order to help Donny continue to work on his Irrational Beliefs between sessions; thus, change will likely occur more quickly.

Session 2:

Analysis: During the first session the therapist introduced the ABC Model and spoke about Irrational Beliefs and how they impact emotions. The D, E and F of the ABC Model was not discussed early on because it is often not addressed until later sessions. During this session the therapist will begin to help Donny learn how to combat those Irrational Beliefs on his own, so that he is not dependent on a therapist to improve his emotional status.

T – It is good to see you. How did things go this week?

DK – Things suck. You should see what my teacher did to my homework this week!

T – Why don't you tell me about it.

DK – I did all of this work on it. It was more like a project then a paper and I can't even tell why I got the F. Take a look at it! I brought it with me so you can see I am not lying.

T – (Therapist flips through homework) I can see your frustration. There really isn't much feedback to work with here. By any chance did you do your therapy homework about this situation this week?

DK – Yes, I even wrote it down.

T – [Slight Laughter] Good. Can I see it?

DK – I didn't bring it.

T – Do you remember what you wrote down about it?

DK – [Slight Chuckle] Of course I brought it. I actually wrote it down. I wanted to show you what I did. I want to know what you think about my writing.

Analysis: At this point Donny still exhibits Irrational Thinking. He desires the therapist's approval. This exhibits the Irrational Belief that we must be liked by all those around us. It is important for the therapist to try to show Donny that he does not need other's approval in order to be happy.

T – This looks great! It's legible. It looks like you put some real thought into this.

DK – Thanks

T – I see that your teacher gave you a bad grade and you became angry. You ranked yourself an 8 out of ten.

DK – Of course he made me angry. He's interfering with my chance to go to college.

T – Let's back up for a moment. You made yourself angry.

> *Analysis:* Here the therapist is helping the client to identify what they are doing to create their own stress in life. By utilizing confrontation, the therapist is trying to get Donny to take responsibility for his own IB. The method of confrontation used here is more forceful than other therapeutic techniques.

DK- Right, I made myself angry [Sarcasm is in his voice]. That stupid should!

> *Analysis:* The fact that Donny utilizes the word should shows that he is beginning to understand where his feelings are coming from. This is a good sign that he will be able to internalize the process of REBT and become independent in disputing his own negative feelings.

T - Is this the same teacher we talked about last week?

DK – Of course it is. We all hate him. Here, take a look at this homework assignment. Now tell me why I got a bad grade. Look at all the work I put into that. [Donny pulls the homework assignment out of his brief case].

T – Oh, I can see why you are frustrated. I am not sure why you got a bad grade either. The teacher did not say much on this assignment to help you understand.

DK – See! I think the teacher should grade me on my mechanical abilities, ya know, my actual work on a car.

T – I know that you can restate that sentence. You did it in your therapeutic homework. Why don't you do it now.

> *Analysis:* The reason the therapist is making Donny restate the sentence is because he will not be able to change his depressive thinking until he can begin to let go of his Irrational Beliefs and replace them with Rational Beliefs.

DK – It would be really beneficial if my teacher would grade me on my actual mechanical abilities instead of what I can put on paper. (Sarcasm in his voice)

T – There you go. You did it. If you think about it that way, then does your rating change in regards to your anger?

DK – Maybe I'm not as angry, but it is really frustrating that I can't show anyone what I know because they only want it on paper.

T – So let's talk about that. It is frustrating to you that you can't show people what you know, the way you want to. What other emotions do you feel about that?

DK – Hopeless, depressed. I have always had learning difficulty, but mechanics is my strength, what I'm good at. Now, since starting with this teacher I am starting to think that I'm not as good as I thought I was. I don't know what I'm going to do if I don't work on cars. I'm worthless. Or I feel like I'm becoming worthless. I don't know.

T – All right. There are 2 pieces to this conversation. First, we need to think about why people become depressed. Second, we need to identify possible careers that do not require a college degree. That piece can be part of your homework. So, let's talk about why people become depressed. There are 3 primary reasons for the depression. First, a person may blame themselves thinking that they are causing the depression. Second you may be having a pity party for yourself. Third you may be having a pity party for someone else. So that means you may feel bad about some else's problems. As you think about them, it disturbs you that you can't help them. It sounds to me that you are feeling sorry for yourself because you are thinking "poor me" I will never grow up and make anything of my life. I'm not getting anywhere. I feel sorry for myself because everyone else thinks I'm stupid. Right? When thinking about your depression or hopelessness, does that make sense? Correct me if I'm wrong.

> *Analysis:* The word hopeless during a therapeutic session should not be taken lightly. Here, the therapist is choosing to hone in on Donny's problem of depression, not the activating events that he Irrationally Believes are the reason for his depression. Donny clearly thinks that he should be good at mechanics and that it is his only way of becoming an independent adult. Consequently, he awfulizes when he gets a bad grade and his opportunity to attend college appears less viable to him. He is unable to see that he has value just because he is a human being. He feels he needs to perform a certain way, and that in doing so everyone should see his intelligence and value him for it.

DK – Wow. I haven't thought about it that way. I feel like my depression comes out of the fact that I'm so frustrated that no one takes me seriously because of my learning disabilities. But maybe I am pitying myself because I don't think anyone takes me seriously. I really just need to think about this. I don't know.

T – This is a great place to stop. You need to go away and think about this. For homework, I want you to do two things. First, I want you to think about what contributes to your depression and challenge those negative thoughts. Second, I want you to write down five careers that do not require a college education.

Session 3:

T - Hi Donny. How are you?

DK – I'm OK.

T – I'm really excited to hear about what you came up with pondering the idea that you are pitying yourself? (therapist says with sideways smile)

> *Analysis*: Humor is a popular technique utilize by REBT therapists to counterattack the over-serious side of individuals.

DK – [Chuckle] I hate to think of it that way, but yay, I think I might be. I feel like I have some real reasons to be upset and frustrated. But if I really think about it, maybe feeling sorry for myself is why I get so angry.

T – What do you really have to pity yourself for?

DK - Excuse me?

T – Are you really someone I should pity?

> *Analysis:* The therapist is choosing to use a functional dispute to encourage the client to start understanding that it is his own irrational belief system that is impacting his thought process and causing him to pity himself.

DK – We talked about this. My teacher thinks I'm stupid. He is failing me on all my written assignments. He could care less what I can do under the hood of the car. If he fails me, I will get kicked out, never graduate from High School, and never be independent enough to leave my parents' house. How am I going to get a job without a college degree? All successful people go to college. All I see when I look around my town are professionals. What's wrong with me? Why can't I even write a simple sentence correctly? Why does everyone else have it so easy?

T – It sounds like you are blaming yourself for not living up to your own standards so you feel inadequate.

DK – Well, who else's fault can it be? I'm the one with the learning disability. But why did God make me this way?

T – Let's talk about what your standards are for yourself. Maybe they are not realistic. What would life look like for you in ten years if you had no problems in school?

> *Analysis:* The therapist is moving towards an empirical disputation. By helping Donnie develop a more rational belief system the therapist is guiding him toward new and healthy feelings.

DK – I'd have a college degree, a great paying job, a house, a wife and some kids [chuckle]. I'd be in a great neighborhood where my kids could go out on the street and play. They would have a great public education. My mom and dad would be proud of me. My sisters would have someone to look up to. I'd be like the rest of my friends. Who wants to marry someone who can't support themselves?

T- Those sounds like great goals. Why do you think you need a college education to attain those them? We do need to be realistic. Maybe you don't have the aptitude to go for college. Why frustrate yourself trying to get there? You have to be aware of your own strengths and use them to meet realistic goals. Your goals are not unrealistic. The way you want to get there may be. Do you know anyone who is successful who did not attend college?

> *Analysis:* The therapist is trying to move Donny toward self-acceptance by helping him understand that he, like others, has both strengths and weaknesses. If he can accept his weaknesses then he is able to focus his attention on his strengths and utilize them to attain his goals, instead of focusing on his weaknesses and pitying himself. This self-acceptance is a healthier and more rational way of thinking, which will ultimately lead to positive self-efficacy.

DK – [Chuckle] Jimi Hendrix. He was an amazing musician making a ton of money. Anyone would have married him!

T – So let's set some goals for you. They need to be realistic, utilize your aptitudes, and help you obtain the goals you are talking about. There is a benefit to not going to college. You are going to start making money right away and you will not be building debt. Let's think about these two guys. The first one goes to law school and the other one starts working right away. First, law school takes about three years after going to college. That is essentially 7 years of schooling. Assuming you don't have any debt from college, you are going to come out of law school with about $100,000 that you have to pay back. Then you likely have to take a job that you aren't thrilled about, with very long hours, working for someone else just to make enough money to live and pay back debt. On the other hand, let's think about the other guy who starts working right away. While he may start out as low man on the totem pole, he may very well be in management by the time the other guy graduates from law school; with no debt. The person in law school likely doesn't own a house and getting a loan for one could prove difficult because he has a huge debt hanging over his head. The guy working has likely saved up for a down payment on a house and may actually own one by now.

> *Analysis:* The REBT Therapist does not hesitate to be directive toward the client. The goal is to be quick and efficient in helping the client change their irrational belief system. That is why homework is utilized as a means in assisting the client understand the nature of the problem.

DK – Silence

T – These guys both chose career goals that played to their strengths. The Lawyer probably argues well, but couldn't fix a car if he had to. The Mechanic may well be a nice guy who is a little introverted, but runs circles around the Lawyer under the hood of a car.

> *Analysis*: This is a philosophical disputation. Donny is determining that he will only be successful if he goes to college. The therapist is utilizing a philosophical dispute in order to get him to understand that he is able to choose a different path and he will still be a success. Donny's belief of the need to go to college is supported by the cultural norms.

DK – I'm not introverted!

T and DK – [share a laugh]

DK – That is a good point. I never looked at it that way. I guess I do need to recognize that I have some strengths.

> *Analysis:* The disputations utilized so far appear to be effective with Donny, as he is beginning to recognize that his weaknesses do not have to be the focus of his thinking. The therapist wants to guide Donny in a manner that helps foster self-acceptance.

T – This is a perfect time to talk about the homework we had you do last week where we asked you to list careers that don't require a college education.

DK – Well, you are right, a mechanic doesn't need a college degree. My friend mentioned that his dad is a carpenter and doesn't have a degree. I like to weld. I could do that. Plumbers, pipe fitters, being a restaurant manager, or being a landscaper don't really require a degree. My sister's Godmother told me that I could even be a pharmacy tech without a degree from college. Can you imagine that? I can hand out drugs!

T – So do you think those people go on to get married and have kids?

DK – Probably. And if I worked as a pharmacy tech people would probably think that I did have a degree.

T – OK, so maybe you don't need that college degree that has been hanging over your head. Next week when we meet, let's talk about some goals to get you where you want to go.

Session 4:

T – Hi Donny. How are you today?

DK – Doing better.

T – Great! What do you think is the reason you are doing better?

> *Analysis:* The therapist is attempting to determine if Donny is internalizing REBT Therapy since he reports that he is feeling better.

DK – It seems like maybe there is a future for me. Maybe I can actually have that normal life with a wife and kids.

T – Wonderful. I wanted to talk to you about the process of obtaining those goals. Let's talk about what a SMART Goal is. SMART stands for specific, measurable, attainable, realistic, and time bound. I thought we would take a small goal you have and work through it so that you understand how to write a goal like this. What do you think?

> *Analysis:* The therapist is once again being directive in an effort to keep Donny focused on his rational thought processes. Goal setting is frequently utilized in many different therapeutic approaches.

DK – Sure. Sounds complicated. Do I have to write it down?

T – I think it would be good. The only person who has to refer back to it and read it from time to time is you. As long as you know what you wrote down it doesn't matter if anyone else can read it. So, what is one goal that you want to work on.

DK – I want a good job, a house, a wife and kids.

T – That is a broad goal that will take a long time to accomplish. It will take a lot of smaller goals that have a more specific end date to get there. Keep the broad goal in mind and let's start working on the small steps that will get you there.

DK – I want to pass this mechanics class!

T – Great! We can work with that.

DK – Well, I want to pass this class, but the teacher is really down on everything that I do. I never pass the exams even when I know how to do all of the technical work. So how are you going to help me accomplish that?

T – Good question. I'm going to hand you this sheet and we are going to walk through it together. You can write on this sheet and I'll give you a clean copy to take home so that you can refer to it in the future. The first question is, what do you want to accomplish at this time?

> *Analysis:* While REBT therapy does not have a specific template required for goal setting; they do find it to be a beneficial activity. Most of the reason goals aren't accomplished is because clients don't know how to be specific or are typically too vague when setting goals. Therefore, utilizing SMART goals gives the client the framework to write a successful goal.

DK – I already told you. I want to pass this class.

T – Let's start with the S; which stands for specific. Who will be a part of you accomplishing this goal?

DK – My sister and my parents and maybe some classmates.

T – What is required to accomplish this goal?

DK – We aren't getting anywhere. I already told you this. I don't know what I can do to pass this class. I've thought of everything, I've tried everything, and I'm still failing.

T – I understand that. But what grade do you need to get in order to pass this class? You need to think more specifically. Break it down to identify a specific goal. We aren't going to revert back to being negative and having a pity party. So, what grade do you need to get?

> *Analysis:* Therapist is being directive and requiring empirical evidence for his irrational belief to keep him from falling into his negative thought process.

DK – [eye roll] For this school I need to get a C. If I were anywhere else a 'D' would work. But I need to maintain a specific grade point average to stay in this school.

T – So what can you do to get a 'C' in the class? Think in terms of what actions you need to do. I'm thinking about homework assignments, tests, participation grades, things like that.

DK – I have four projects due this month and have to get an 'A' or a 'B' on those projects. I am failing now so if I were to get a 'B' then I would probably be able to pass.

T – Great! Where would this goal be accomplished?

DK – Are you serious? What do you mean by where? At school. That's where I would do my work. Where else do you do classwork? [Pause] Oh yeah, I guess you could do it at home.

T – Why do you want to accomplish this goal?

DK – I want to make money and live on my own!

T – When would you accomplish this goal?

DK – Excuse me?

T – For instance, now, next week, over the next year.

DK – I need to accomplish this by the end of the semester.

T – Ok, how many weeks do you have left in this semester?

DK – We are four weeks into the semester and I have about 8 weeks left. So, when I think about it, I actually have some time. I kind of get where you are coming from now. It seems a little more manageable.

T – Okay. Let's get a little more specific. Each project needs to get done in about a week and a half. Do you think you can do that?

DK – If my sister helps me then yes, I think I can do it.

> *Analysis:* The therapist is utilizing Socratic dialogue by which she is acting as the facilitator and asking Donny guiding questions that he has to answer. By doing this the

> therapist is guiding his thought process and trying to elicit certain responses in accordance with identifying goals.

T – Great! Let's move on. A stands for attainable. What we are really trying to get at is, are there resources within your environment available to help you attain this goal? Do you know what resources are necessary?

> *Analysis:* In REBT the therapist often moves the session along quickly to keep the client focused forward. It is harder for a client to have a pity party if the therapist questions the client in almost a rapid-fire manner.

DK – Resources? You mean like a pen and paper?

T – Yes, I'm thinking tangible things. But I'm also thinking about resources like tutoring. Do you have access to those resources?

DK – Yes, my mom and dad can get me a tutor, but my sister does that for me too. But I try not to use my sister as much. She is in high school too and I want her to be able to get her work done. So maybe I can ask my parents to get me a tutor for the next 8 weeks.

T – Great! Then do you think that this goal is attainable?

DK – Yes.

T – Next, we are going to talk about whether the goal is realistic or not.

DK – What, you don't think I can do it? I'm nothing if not realistic.

T – [Laughs] It's the R in SMART goals Donny. Do you have time to accomplish this goal?

DK – I think so; especially since we just talked about me having a week and a half to accomplish these projects. I may have to take a day or two off from work; however.

T – Okay. So how will accomplishing this goal affect you?

DK – Are you kidding. I'll actually get to stay in school and my parents may not have to let me live with them for the rest of my life.

T – Well, you actually just answered the next question. This goal seems to have a positive impact on your entire family. So, do you think that this goal is realistic?

DK – Yes.

T – Finally, the last part. T stands for time-bound. That means, when will you accomplish this goal?

DK – By the end of the semester. Obviously.

T – Are there things that may get in the way of you accomplishing this goal by the end of the semester?

DK – Well, there is my teacher who would love to fail me. So, he could get in the way. Also, my tutor has to understand what I am working on. Not everyone understands mechanics.

T – That's a great point. See you have a lot of value. Ok, with all of this information, we are going to be more specific about your goal.

DK – This is a lot of work.

T – Yes, but the point is that you have to overcome the way you look at things. This is what I'm talking about. The actual goal is: to pass your mechanics class in the next 8 weeks. You accomplish this by getting a grade of 'B' or higher on the next 5 projects utilizing a tutor educated in mechanics. Can you see how this goal is more useful than saying that 'I just want to pass this class?'

DK – Yes but I'm not understanding what you mean when you say that I have to overcome the way I look at things.

T – Remember what we discussed the first time we met? That we have rational and irrational beliefs. An irrational belief causes your own distress. We talked about the ways in which you are depressing yourself. Whenever I listen to you, you are putting more value on what others think of you then what you think of yourself. In doing this, you tend to awfulize situations. What do you think about that?

> *Analysis*: Donny still has a habit of thinking that outside forces cause his Depression. The therapist is reminding him, that it is his thought processes that have this effect. When Donny focuses outward, everything seems awful. A person cannot control what another is doing to them, only what their reaction to the situation is. When Donny focuses on the goal, he stops looking outward to blame others for his current situation.

DK – [Silence].

T – Awfulizing often leads to self-pity. So, the depression that you feel is related to how you are thinking about your teacher and his impact on your life.

DK – Wow! I know we talked about this before. But saying it that way makes sense. I think I kind of get what you mean. I need to overcome how I think about what other people think. Right?

T – Exactly, but let's take it a step further. The rational belief is to determine how you value yourself. It really doesn't matter what other people think about you. These rational thoughts lead to healthier feelings. So, the ultimate goal of REBT isn't to talk out an issue until you are desensitized. It isn't to find diversions to your feelings so you don't feel them. It is to help you learn not to depress yourself even when things go wrong. It is to help you learn to take that irrational thought and determine what makes it irrational, and then find the rational thought in the situation.

DK – I think I get where you are coming from. I need to think about this more.

T – This is a great place to stop our session. I have a sheet of homework for you that will help you start to take your irrational thoughts and find the more rational thought process. I want you to begin to identify your irrational thinking on your own. This is the only way you can start moving out of your depression.

Session 5:

(During this session, Donny is focusing on his dyslexia. He uses the term to describe both dyslexia and dysgraphia. We are not defining the two in therapy, as this would not necessarily benefit him during this session. Dyslexia refers to reading. Dysgraphia refers to writing.)

T – Hi Donny. How are you doing today?

DK – Fine. I did my homework.

T – Can I see it? (Silence while the therapist looks at the homework). Wow Donny, you put a lot of work into this. You have three different examples. Do you feel like you understood the homework?

DK – Yeah. It took a lot of effort though. That's a lot of writing.

T – I understand that, but you did a great job. Which one of these would you like to go over?

DK – Why don't we just look at the first one. If I can't write a receipt for my job, how am I even going to get a job?

> *Analysis:* Donny is overgeneralizing here. The homework helps Donny pinpoint the irrational thought on his own so that he can learn to challenge himself.

T – Well, let's start by pointing out that you have a job. How did you get this particular job?

> *Analysis:* The therapist is using a technique often used in REBT to move the client past their negative thinking. It is called confrontation. The therapist wants to provide the client with the tools to help him change his beliefs as often as possible, so this technique is often used.

DK – My parents know the owner and he offered to give me a job pumping gas. But he also knew that I was interested in mechanics so he started letting me work on cars too.

T – So that is a very legitimate way to get a job. It's called networking. I remember when I was trying to get this job, I let all my old professors know that I was job hunting. One of them sent me a job posting back and told me if I applied, they would put in a good word for me. That is how I got my interview. But let's get back to the homework assignment. What was happening that made you write this down on your homework?

> *Analysis:* The REBT Therapist utilized self-disclosure in this situation to help normalize Donny's experience of getting a job through networking. The therapist is choosing to educate the client to help him dispute the idea that the way he got a job is different from other people. Donny uses language and thinking that is self-defeating and often self-prophesying. This does not help him learn unconditional self-acceptance which is important for Donny to achieve good mental health and reduce his depression.

DK – I was at work and pumping gas. Normally my friend is at work with me and he just writes my receipts, but he was home sick. I had a customer pull up to full service. I went out and pumped his gas and wrote up his receipt and handed it to him. He was frustrated because he couldn't read it. He asked me to rewrite it and he wasn't happy with the second one either. I ended up having to ask one of the mechanics to write it, which frustrates them because it's not their job. I walked away feeling like "if I can't do this, how am I ever going to get a real job, one where I can move out of my parent's house and support myself. I can't even do a basic thing like write a receipt."

T – Donny, stop telling yourself garbage. If you keep telling yourself you are a failure you will fail, not because of your disability, but because you will convince yourself.

> *Analysis:* At this point we are firmly disputing and attacking his beliefs because he needs to learn that he is responsible for his own depressive thinking. This self-prophesying is the main reason for his failure. Instead of coming up with ways to work past his disability, he is staying in a place of self-pity. We want him to learn to dispute his own thinking and accept his disability in an unconditional way.

T – I know you've done this already, but let's go through this sheet. I want to make sure that you understand how to do this for yourself. Our goal is for you to learn how to dispute your own irrational thinking so that you don't always need to be in therapy. Let's look at the first question on your homework sheet. Is there substantial evidence for your thought process? Has it happened before?

> *Analysis:* The therapist is utilizing an empirical dispute when she asks him for substantial evidence for his thought process.

DK – I've always been in luck because my friend is usually at work with me, but anytime he is gone it is going to be a problem. I don't write well. My dyslexia gets in the way. How do you overcome that?

> *Analysis*: Donny continues to be self-defeating and the therapist needs to find a way to confront Donny so that he is able to change his perspective. The goal of the REBT therapist right now is to get the client to be an active participant in life and to use rational

thinking in problem solving.

T - Good question. Write that down. Let's keep going through the sheet and come back to that. Is there any evidence to the contrary?

> *Analysis*: The therapist is keeping Donny on task by not addressing his irrational beliefs at this moment. She is forcing him to continue to show empirical evidence that will ultimately help him move beyond his pattern of negative thinking.

DK – Well, the mechanics don't do their receipts. We have an office manager for them.

T - Oh, that's interesting. Let's jot that down too. So, are you interpreting the situation with all the evidence?

DK – The evidence is that I can't write a receipt.

T – But not everyone writes their own receipt at the shop, right? What other evidence is there that you won't get a job that allows you to move out of the house if you can't write a receipt?

DK – [Chuckle] OK. It's just that if I can't write, I am going to have a problem getting a job.

T – What are some ways to overcome your writing difficulties? Is there anything available to you at the shop that can produce a receipt?

DK – Other than the office manager?

T – [Chuckle] Yes.

DK – Like a computer?

T – Yes! So, six months from now, will it matter if you are able to write a receipt if you can use technology to do the work for you? Or will this matter a year from now?

DK – Maybe not. Hmm.

T – So if you look at the attached sheet, can you figure out which maladaptive thought process that is?

DK – Is it perfectionism or overgeneralizing?

> *Analysis*: The therapist is helping Donny to label the maladaptive thought patterns. When he is able to independently do this, he will be able to identify his own rational thought patterns from the irrational beliefs he has created, and will have a healthier pattern of thinking. This will ultimately allow him to dispute his own depression.

T – Perfectionism is the need to have everything perfect. Do you have a need for the receipt to be perfect? On the other hand, overgeneralizing is when a person takes one bad situation and thinks that it will happen every time or that it will impact everything else.

DK – I don't really care what the receipt looks like. Everyone else seems to care. So, I guess I'm overgeneralizing.

T – Good. Overgeneralizing is an irrational thought process. Can you find the alternative view to this situation that will help you come up with a more rational thought? I know this is kind of complicated so we are going to think about this a little differently. Let's pretend that we are in a court room. The thought is on trial. The defense is evidence for your thought and the prosecution is evidence against the thought. Then we have a verdict and the judge decides if the thought is reasonable or not. You can actually do this every time you have an irrational thought. Let's try thinking about your irrational belief in this way.

> *Analysis:* Here, the therapist is teaching Donny how to utilize logical disputation to change his own perspective. By putting the thought on trial Donny can logically work through whether or not the thought is logical without his ego being involved.

DK – Ok, that's a little clearer. So, you are saying that my thought of never finding a job because I can't write a receipt is on trial.

T – That is exactly what I'm saying. Let's think about the defense's argument first.

DK – Ok, if I were the defense, I would say that it is perfectly reasonable that I will not be able to get a job because I can't write. I would even call the person who couldn't read the receipt as a witness. He told me that the receipt has to be legible because it is a tax write off for his job. I'd also call my boss as a witness. So far, he hasn't really been aware of the problem because my friend was writing the receipt. But, I bet he would say that I need to be able to provide a legible receipt.

T – Maybe. What about for the prosecution? What would they say about the thought that you must write a receipt to get a good job?

DK – I would call my friend who writes the receipts for me. He would say I don't always need to be the one to write them. I wonder what my educational psychologist would say? She is always talking about "reasonable accommodations." I hate that phrase. She might ask about the computer option for doing my job. My boss is pretty cool. If we problem solved this together, he might actually say that since I have an alternative most of the time, maybe the office manager could help on the rare occasion that my friend is not at work.

T – So what do you think the judge is going to say in this particular case?

DK – That is a good question. I guess he might say that with the right accommodations I can get a job that will pay well.

T – So, the rational thought is?

DK – I just said it. With the right accommodations I can get a job that will pay well enough for me to live on my own.

> *Analysis:* Most clients know what their issue is. They can state that they are depressed, that they have anxiety, or that they are neurotic. They just don't have the tools to change their thought patterns. REBT therapists know that if a client can be taught to dispute their own irrational beliefs, then they can be taught to operationally change their thought processes and move beyond their irrational thinking. By teaching Donny to remove himself from the process and only analyze his thoughts, he is able to move toward healthier thinking.

T – Nice job! Now we need to think a little more about rational and irrational thoughts because when I'm not with you it will be important for you to be able to identify when you have an irrational thought. How did you decide what to use on your homework?

DK – Well, I was thinking about what causes me to feel bad, or as you therapists would say "depressed." I don't like feeling that way and some thoughts really contribute to those feelings. That is what I thought of when I was doing the homework. According to you those thoughts are irrational, right?

T - You've got it. So, what makes a thought rational?

DK – It's a little more logical according to your sheet. The rational thought is supported by evidence and is not necessarily based on my feelings.

T – Do you think the homework was helpful, and you would use it outside of session?

> *Analysis*: By assigning homework, the therapist is getting the client to think through and change patterns of thought and subsequent behavior. This specific homework assignment is designed to change Donny's thinking from "can't do" to "can do." By thinking of different ways that he "can do" something, this will empower Donny. The therapist would like for Donny to change his thinking and to show him that risk-taking is not catastrophic, and that he has some ideas that will motivate change from irrational thinking.

DK – Well how long would I have to do this homework?

T – The goal is that by using this worksheet, it will help you to make irrational thinking more rational. It is just one coping skill in your bag of tricks, the judge and jury is another one. I want you to be able to identify when you are starting to feel depressed. Think about what irrational thoughts you have that contribute to your depression, and start to think about it in a rational way. So, you don't have to use this homework every day. It's just one of many coping skills that you now have to dispute your thinking. How often you use it depends on how often it helps you work through irrational thinking.

DK – So you're saying that I don't always have to use the worksheet, but it is a tool that I can use to help me get rid of those negative thoughts.

T – Those irrational thoughts.

DK – I mean, those irrational thoughts. I think I can do that.

T – Let's go two weeks between the next session. I'm here if you need me, don't hesitate to call. But I want to see if this is something you can do for yourself and if you can use these skills in your everyday life.

DK – See you in two weeks.

Session 6:

T - So, I didn't get a call or a text or a message from the answering service. How did you do? Did you white knuckle it to this appointment, or did you find the skills we have been working on helpful?

DK – Actually, I think I did pretty well. I mainly used that rational/irrational thinking stuff. I really like the judge and jury way of thinking about things. I even used it on my little sister.

T – On your little sister, huh? For what?

DK – She was going to quit dance and I don't think she should. So, we played judge and jury. I think that I am really getting the hang of doing this for myself. I actually feel pretty good about it. I've been in therapy my whole life and I want to give this a shot by myself.

T – You mean you want this be your last session?

DK – Yes.

T – I'm game, as long as you promise to call if it's not working. Think of this like a vaccination. Sometimes you need a booster shot. I'm going to give you a book of worksheets to take with you too. You can always call and ask about any of these sheets if you want to implement a new one to help you out.

DK – I think having resources available to me will be helpful.

T – Good. Let's make sure you are really ready for this to be your last session. Do you remember us talking about the A-B-C model?

DK – Vaguely. Is that when there is something that happens that causes me to believe something. Then how I behave is the consequence?
T – That's it.

DK – I remember that because we were talking about that shop teacher I don't like very much.

And I thought that I was getting in trouble because the guy just didn't like me, but I realized that walking out of class did not help my situation.

T – Good. Now do you remember the 3 reasons for depression?

DK – Are you quizzing me right now? You know my feelings about quizzes, right?

T – Yes, aren't you happy that this is an oral exam?

DK – A person can be depressed because they blame themselves, they are having a pity party, or they feel pity for someone else.

T – You are on a roll. Do you remember the SMART goals we talked about?

DK – I have a sheet for that one.

T – Will you remember to use it?

DK – Yes. That one was actually helpful.

T – Ok, can you tell me the difference between rational and irrational beliefs?

DK – An irrational thought is something that doesn't have evidence and is based more on my feelings than on logic. A rational thought has evidence to support it,, and supports healthy thinking.

T – Ok, you have the gist of everything we discussed. Let's get back to that promise that you will come back to see me if you are having a hard time with your irrational beliefs.

DK – I will.

T – Actually I need you to say 'I promise that I will come back if I'm starting to become depressed or if I need help with the homework sheets.'

DK – [eye roll]. Ok, I promise that I will come back if I'm starting to become depressed or need help with my homework sheets.

T – Great! I am excited for you. What are you going to do with the extra hour a week you have on your hands?

DK – I'm going to work on my homework.

T – Sounds like a great plan. Here is my business card in case you don't have one. Carry it in your wallet and call me anytime.

DK – Thank you. I promise I will.

Analysis: The goal of therapy was to help Donny reduce his depressive symptoms by helping him understand how his irrational thinking was facilitating his depression. The therapist was able to provide Donny with concrete ways to dispute his irrational thought processes. He is now able to utilize homework sheets and alternative coping skills to move toward more rational and self-accepting thoughts. Donny is aware he can return at any time should the need arise, but feels ready to move toward more healthy thinking on his own for now. Therefore, the goals of therapy have been met.

References

Capuzzi, D., & Gross, D. R. (2007). *Counseling and psychotherapy: Theories and interventions* (4th ed.). New Jersey: Pearson Education Inc.

Corey, G. (1996). *Theory and practice of counseling and psychotherapy* (5th ed.). Pacific Grove, CA: Brooks/Cole Publishing Company.

Corsini, R. J., & Wedding, D. (2005). *Current psychotherapies* (7th ed.). Belmont, CA: Brooks/Cole Publishing Company.

Corsini, R.J. & Wedding, D. (2019). *Current psychotherapies* (11th ed.). Boston, MA: Cengage Learning, Inc.

DiGiuseppe, R. (1999). End piece: Reflections on the treatment of anger. *Journal of Clinical Psychology, 55*(3), 365-379.

Ellis, A. (2004). *Rational emotive behavior therapy: It works for me-it can work for you.* Amherst, NY: Prometheus Books.

Ellis, A., & Harper, R. A. (1997). *A guide to rational living.* North Hollywood, CA: Melvin Powers.

Ellis, A & MacLauren, C. (2005). *Rational emotive behavior therapy: A therapists guide* (2nd ed.). Atascadero, CA: Impact Publishers.

Jones, R. G. (1969). *A factored measure of Ellis' irrational belief system, with personality and maladjusted correlates* [Dissertation, Texas Technical College]. https://ttu-ir.tdl.org

Thompson, C. L., & Rudolph, L. B. (1999). *Counseling children* (5th ed.). Pacific Grove, CA: Brooks/Cole Publishing Company.

Wedding, D., & Corsini, R. J. (2019). *Current Psychotherapies* (11th ed.). Boston, MA: CENGAGE Learning, Inc.

SECTION III: Adlerian Therapy

History of the Founder

Alfred Adler was born in Penzing, a suburb of Vienna, Austria, on February 7, 1870. His father was a corn-merchant who took pride in his shrewd business acumen that allowed him to provide generously for his family at the time of Alfred's birth. Alfred inherited, or "chose" (Bottome, 1939) to emulate his father's happy disposition and spiritual qualities. His mother was often described as moody and nervous, which contributed to the strained relationship between them. Alfred's family included three brothers, himself, and two sisters (Bottome, 1939), not counting two that died in infancy. Coming from a large family, he felt overshadowed by a "model" eldest brother (Bottome, 1939), who always seemed to out-perform him in all endeavors. However, as they grew older, Alfred spoke of his eldest brother with reverence and admiration. The third brother, born after Alfred, was often jealous of Alfred's popularity. This contributed to a strained relationship throughout life. Richard was the youngest brother and born at a time when the family was thrust into sudden poverty. While his older siblings had enjoyed a prosperous childhood, the poverty of his parent's made education and prospects bleak for Richard. Being Alfred's favorite, Richard was doted on materially and spiritually by Alfred all his life. Alfred had good relationships with his two sisters, especially during early childhood and managed to keep in touch with them throughout adulthood. It is from this perspective that he was able to develop his ideas of birth order later on.

Alfred was a youth in the 1880's when Vienna was a luxurious and modern city standing at the peak of European civilization. On summer evenings, Alfred's family and friends would often meet at their favorite vineyard, to eat, drink, and sing. According to Bottome (1939), Alfred would often take part in the signing and he enjoyed playing accompaniments on the piano with his younger sister Hermine. While music was a lingering passion, school was not. He achieved only mediocrity in school, failing mathematics at one point, and having to repeat the class. His teachers did not have much confidence in his academic abilities. On one occasion, a teacher even told Alfred's father that Alfred should be a shoemaker (Corey 1996). This appears to have given Adler the determination to do better, as he eventually rose to the top of his class.

Alfred had always intended to be a doctor. He attended college at the Medical School of the University of Vienna, where he was able to hold his own among peers. During his time at the university, Adler mastered the history of psychology and began to form an opinion upon which the rest of his career was based. The end of Alfred's university career was hampered by his lack of resources (Bottome, 1939) and by falling in love with Raissa Timofejewna. Raissa was born in Moscow to wealthy parents, and her uncle owned several railway lines (Bottome, 1939). She was educated and was an expert translator. She had a natural talent for writing. Alfred and Rassia were married in 1897, two years after he graduated from the university. They had four children: Valentine, Alexandra, Kurt and Cornelia.

In the early days of marriage, Alfred worked as a general practitioner of medicine and served as a physician for the Hungarian Army. From his student days, he was linked to the cause of social betterment. He wrote a pamphlet entitled The Health of Taylors; discussing the conditions of Taylor shops in Vienna. It is around this time that Freud's famous book on Dream Analysis was published. While Freud's book was widely ridiculed among Viennese medical circles, Alfred wrote a strong defense of the book. Freud was touched by Adler's stance and sent him a postcard asking him to join his discussion group called the "Wednesday Society" (Capuzzi & Gross, 2007). This later became the spring board of the psychoanalytic movement.

Differing ideas and viewpoints ultimately caused a rift between Freud and Adler. The year 1910 was considered Alfred Alder's launch into freedom as he was no longer in the shadow of Freud. He gave up his general practice entirely and devoted himself to the practice of psychiatry. In 1911, Adler gave up his post as president of the Vienna Psychoanalytic Society and in 1912, he founded the Society for Free Psychoanalytic Research (Corsini & Wedding, 1995).

In 1922, Alfred created child-guidance clinics in the Vienna public schools and trained professionals such as teachers, social workers, and physicians on how to work with children (Corey, 1996; Mosak, 1995). He set up 28 clinics to be overseen by psychologists who volunteered their time. It is around this time that Alfred also traveled between the United States and Vienna. In the United States he served for the Medical Faculty of the Long Island College of Medicine. In 1934 when a fascist government shut down his clinics in Vienna, he moved to the U.S. for good. He died of a heart attack in Aberdeen, Scotland while taking a walk before a scheduled lecture on May 28, 1937.

Due to Alfred's success with Child Guidance Clinics inside the Vienna school system, Rudolf Dreikurs decided to follow his model and bring these clinics into the United States. The success of the schools in the United States prompted the Vienna School System to invite Adlerian Psychotherapists back into the country to plan and open a school that emphasized encouragement, class discussion, democratic principles, and responsibility (Mosak, 1995).

Contrasting REBT to Adlerian Therapy
What Ellis called Irrational Beliefs; Adler calls basic mistakes. Both theories believe that in order to control emotions, one must first control their thought processes. This allows us to be creators of our emotions instead of victims of them (Mosak, 1995).

Construct of Personality

Adler believed that all behavior happens in social context. We are born into a family and engage into reciprocal relationships. In fact, Adlerian Therapy believes that people cannot be studied in isolation. Adler himself was quoted to say "in the history of human civilization, no form of life whose foundations were not laid communal can be found" (Adler, 2010, p. 28). It is in this context of relationship that a person develops their lifestyle, or way of perceiving and responding to the world.

Early Childhood Development

Every person is born into a family or social system. Typically, the family is the first social group for a child. In the case of an orphan, the orphanage becomes their family. It is within this context that the child begins to make assumptions about who they are. They develop ideas about how the world functions, how it treats them, and how others treat them. For instance, if a child is born into a hostile home, they will likely decide that the world is hostile. However, it is important to understand that each person is different and will interpret their experiences in their own unique way. What one child perceives as hostile, another child might perceive as an everyday occurrence. It is also important to understand that as the family system changes, a child's perception can change. Therefore, when another child is born, the oldest child may feel displaced, or may enjoy the new experience of being an older sibling. Age difference and gender can be an influence on how the other siblings perceive the new child.

Birth Order

Adler felt that birth order had an impact on a child's development. However, it must be understood in the context of the child's social system. Social systems might include the nuclear family. It can also include aunts, uncles, grandparents, or close friends. There do appear, however, to be certain characteristics associated with birth order.

Only children – Only children tend to be unique because they do not have any competition for parental attention. They grow up trying to achieve adult status and often believe that they should have the same status as their parents. Because of this, they often become discouraged and look for alternate ways to be successful, such as being very good at misbehaving. It is the lack of belief that they can become independent and responsible, like their parents, that leads them to find an alternative way to be successful. On the other hand, if given too much attention, they can become helpless as a way of maintaining their parent's attention. Also, because of the lack of sibling rivalry, they do not learn to share their parents or their resources. They rarely need to cooperate with others. Because of their status, they are often valued for just existing. When they develop a talent, they expect the world to recognize and honor that talent. This occurs because they are used to being the center of attention in their home, and are often over recognized for their work inside their social system. Only children can become ego centric and isolated because they perceive their peers to be adults, and are therefore lacking in appropriate peer relationships.

Oldest Children – These children have some period of time being an only child. When the second child comes along the oldest child often feels displaced. In an effort to become special again, they become ultra-responsible. If this does not work, then they may try to become the best in the family at misbehaving. Gender issues can arise based on whether or not the second child is a male or female. For instance, if the first child is a boy and the second child is a girl, she may become daddy's little princess, thereby increasing the feelings of displacement. Whereas if the second child is a boy, then it may be easier for the first child to gain success due to the child's overall maturation both physically and mentally. The older child tends to be responsible, have a good work ethic, and often strives to keep ahead of the rest of his siblings and peers.

The Second Born – They often struggle to find their place in the family. The second child often perceives themselves to be competing with the older child. They desire to surpass their sibling's success. In order to do this, they often find and exploit the older child's weakness in order to gain status in their parent's eyes. However, if the older child is easily able to find success in society and in the family system, then the younger child often becomes quickly discouraged and begins to develop skills that are opposite of the first. For instance, if the older child is good at sports, the younger child may develop talent in art.

The Middle Child – The middle child has a unique position of having a sibling who is ahead of them, as well as a sibling who is trying to catch up with them. Because they are not only trying to catch up to the older child, but are also trying to stay ahead of the younger child they often feel unsure of their place. These children often have low self-esteem, and in order to find a place in the home become the peacemakers of the family.

The Youngest Child – The baby tends to be pampered the most. Since their siblings are always ahead of them, they often beat to their own drum and find their own way in life. Because everyone does everything for them, they often have a hard time developing a sense of responsibility. No matter how capable the youngest child is, they are often not taken seriously because of their status as the baby. The lack of expectation placed on them by the family system, often leads them to become the most successful person in the family.

Lifestyle

Adler (1958) noticed that children that came from the same home often differed widely. This led him to recognize that heredity and environment were not the only determinant for how our personality developed. He began to realize that each individual has his or her own subjective view point that colors the way the individual perceives an event. Because children do not have highly developed logical processes, many of their social perspectives contain errors or partial truths. Due to this personal perspective, Adlerians believe that early memories can help a therapist understand an adult client's perception.

Adler perceived each human being to have an individual lifestyle that refers to one's orientation towards life. Lifestyle includes one's personality, aspirations, and goals that are a requisite for the individual to feel secure and cope with the world. Lifestyle is a primarily unconscious process that includes the cognitive organization of the individual rather than the behavioral. Within this lifestyle one can either behave in a useful or useless manner. When an individual is useful, he or she is wanting to contribute to society and the greater good. Conversely, a useless individual is self-centered and striving only for their own superiority.

Lifestyle can often be divided into four groups: self-concept, self-ideal, world view (*Weltbild*), and ethical convictions (Mosak, 1995). An individual's self-concept refers to how one thinks about themself, and the self-ideal is the individual's beliefs of who they should be. The world view is how we perceive the world around us and what it demands of us. The ethical convictions are our view of what is right and what is wrong. When there is a discrepancy between self-concept and self-ideal, feelings of inferiority begin to develop. Adlerian therapy focuses on these feelings. Such feelings can either motivate humans or discourage goal attainment. By the age of six, it is believed that our self-image is solidified. We begin our life goal of striving to overcome weakness and feelings of inferiority to ultimately become a healthy and functioning member of society. One of the things that led to the rift between Freud and Adler was Adler's perception of feelings of inferiority. For example, Freud thought that women had penis envy whereas Adler simply believed that women had a desire to be equal to, or be respected, as much as men. From an Adlerian perspective, our awareness of being part of a community facilitates our development of social interest. Social interest involves a person figuring out where they belong in their community, and how to contribute to it. It requires an individual to develop empathy. Adler believed that the degree to which we learn to share with others and are concerned for others' welfare, is a measure of mental health (Sherman & Dinkmeyer, 1987 in Mosak, 1995). Adler believed that those who develop social interest become less isolated, where as those who do not develop social interest become discouraged. More recently, Mosak (1977) talked about 5 life tasks that must be confronted and understood in order to be healthy and develop a sense of belonging. These tasks include: "relating to others (friendships), making a contribution (work), achieving intimacy (love and family relationships), getting along with ourselves (self-acceptance), and developing our spiritual dimension (including values, meaning, life goals, and our relationship with the universe, or cosmos)" (Mosak, 1995, p. 138).

"In light of this, part of the therapeutic process requires educating the patient on the following points (Mosak, 1995):

- Fostering social interest
- The decrease of inferior feelings, the overcoming of discouragement, and the recognition and utilization of one's resources.
- Changes in the person's life-style (ie…perceptions and goals).
- Changing faulty behaviors that underlie all behavior, or changing values.
- Encouraging the individual to recognize equality among people (Dreikurs, 1971)
- Helping the person to become a contributing human being"

Once the education process is complete, the patient can then decide to choose self-interest or social- interest based on their updated knowledge. The patient who chooses social-interest experiences a sense of belonging, greater acceptance of self, a greater acceptance of others, and more control over their own destiny. This leads a patient to feel more positive, confident, and encouraged about their life and their future.

Techniques and Procedures

There are four phases or objectives utilized in Adlerian therapy. Just as in life, the stages of therapy are not linear. Clients will move in and out of the different objectives depending on what they are dealing with in the therapeutic session. "The phases include:
1. Establishing the proper therapeutic relationship
2. Discovering the psychological dynamics of the client (analysis and assessment)
3. Encouraging the development of self-understanding (insight)

4. Helping the client make new choices (reorientation and reeducation)" (Corey, 1996).

Phase 1: Establishing the Client/Counselor Relationship

Adlerian's believe that it is important to the therapeutic relationship to establish rapport through collaboration with the client. They recognize the power of empathy in creating a good therapeutic relationship and spend much of their time in the first phase attending and listening. This allows them to identify and clarify goals. Adlerian counselors emphasize the necessity of attending to both verbal and nonverbal cues (e.g., tone of voice, posture, facial expression, etc.) of the client. This permits the counselor to begin to grasp what the client is experiencing, and understand the client's subjective view.

The client-counselor relationship emphasizes the development of rapport through encouragement. Encouragement is both a therapeutic technique as well as way to interact with the client. Focusing on encouragement and identifying strengths or assets leads to a natural break down of a negative self-view. Counselors are future focused and only spend enough time in the past to understand the client's subjective perception. This allows them to determine how to set goals.

Some examples of questions a therapist might ask in an initial session are:
- Do you know why you are here today? (good question for kids)
- Have you ever done therapy before?
- Why did you decide to start therapy?
- How would your life improve if you did not have this problem?

Phase 2: Discovering a Client's Psychological Dynamics

The second phase of therapy is focused on helping the client make a paradigm shift. The client often enters therapy with a very narrow view of their life, which leads to being overwhelmed by even small problems. The counselors' job is to broaden their view and help them understand that their problems can be managed. Adlerian therapists find patterns of faulty behavior that persist in the past and present and will likely impact a client's future. "In order to gain a sense of a client's lifestyle, counselors pay close attention to feelings, motives, beliefs, and goals" (Corey, 1996). By exploring a client's feelings, the counselor can better understand underlying motives for faulty behavior and errors in thinking. Part of the lifestyle assessment includes: looking at the family constellation, listening to early recollections, discussing recurrent dreams, and identifying the client's priorities. The reason for this is to understand the client's interpretation of themselves in a social context as it developed during childhood. Private logic is often uncovered during this process. By understanding these things, it helps the counselor discern how the client is functioning with regards to the life tasks of love, work, friendship, and community. "Adlerian counselors are especially interested in learning about the ways in which the individual meets the basic demands of life" (Corey, 1996, p.45).

Early Recollections: Adlerians utilize early recollections to help them understand the environment in which the client was raised. This is useful information because lifestyles are developed in the first six years of life. Early recollections tend to contain information about the essential beliefs of the client, including what basic mistakes they have established.

Early recollections must be about a specific moment in time. They should be vivid and clear in the mind of the client. When asked about an early recollection, people often give a report of a common occurrence, such as "we use to have dinner with the family every Sunday afternoon." The client must be encouraged at this point to remember a specific point in time. The client may be worried about providing an early memory if he is not sure if it happened or not. However, as long as the memory is vivid, the emotions contained within the memory are intact, and the client remembers details, it does not matter if the memory is real, because it has still helped shape their lifestyle and is important to the therapist's assessment.

When the client provides his or her recollection is important for the therapist to observe and identify the feelings associated with the memory. This allows the therapist to determine how the client perceives themselves. Do they see the world as safe or unsafe? Do they quantify life as fair or unfair? Do they perceive others as being friendly or unfriendly? These early recollections along with family constellation, dreams, and priorities are utilized to understand the client's current lifestyle.

Family Constellation: Adlerians explore family constellations. The purpose is to evaluate the environment during the client's childhood, when a person develops lifestyle convictions and faulty assumptions. Of particular use during this phase is a life-style assessment questionnaire. Mosak and Shulman (1998) *NEED REFERENCE* developed the questionnaire which identified influential factors within the client's life. (See Appendix for an example of a Lifestyle Questionnaire). Some factors include birth order, parent's age at birth, and role in sibling relationships. Once all of the family information has been gathered and the family constellation has been developed, the therapist makes a brief summary on how this information impacts the client's lifestyle.

Dreams: Adler did not believe in fixed symbolism. Instead, he felt that dreams were important to analyze from the perspective of what the client was working through at that point in time. Thus, when analyzing dreams, an Adlerian therapist might examine only pieces of it, in context of what is currently happening. Since Adler viewed behavior as a function of control, power, and motivation, dreams are a way for people to overcompensate for shortcomings during waking hours.

Priorities. Alfred Adler himself did not speak about priorities. He talked about typologies which were his way of differentiating between feelings and behavior. He felt that typologies and lifestyle were the two important things for a therapist to understand about their client in order to best serve them in a therapeutic session. Nira Kfir, an Israeli Psychologist from the Israeli Adlerian Institute in Telaviv, took typologies and extended this idea into personality priorities (Kfir, 2011). She identified four personality priorities that she believes a client uses as their way of coping or belonging. These are the lenses in which you look at the world and how you create an environment that allows you to fit into a social setting.

The four personality priorities that Nera Kfir (Kfir, 2011) identified are: superiority, control, comfort, and pleasing. These are the first lines of defense used by clients when they perceive stress. At times we all use each of these, but during times of crisis most people will default to one primary reaction.

- Superiority – people who default to superiority tend to find their worth in leadership roles and accomplishment. They rarely take part in activities that do not have significance in their eyes. One of the ways to identify a person using this personality priority is that they often report feeling overburdened and overworked.
- Control – people who default to control tend to try to master situations so that they will not be embarrassed in a social situation. These individuals talk about their need to be socially accepted, master situations, and avoid humiliation in public.
- Comfort – people who default to comfort tend to avoid anything that will lead to stressful or painful situations. Such people are identified because they put off making decisions, will constantly report avoidant behaviors, even when the situation is an everyday occurrence.
- Pleasing – people who default to pleasing seek approval constantly. They fear rejection if they are not pleasing others in a social situation. Such people will report going to great lengths for others in order to be accepted, even to the point of burning themselves out at times.

There are two ways to identify what personality priority a client uses most. First, you can ask a client to describe what a typical day looks like. Details such as what they like or dislike about various things they accomplish will provide you with valuable information. Second, you can ask a client to talk about what they avoid doing, why they do so, and what their motive is for avoiding the situation or behavior.

Integration and summary. Once the therapist has gathered information on early recollections, family constellation, dreams, and priorities, this information is summarized and analyzed in conjunction with information from the lifestyle questionnaire. Once the information is summarized, it is discussed with the client and you can begin helping them work through mistakes they have created for themselves.

Phase Three: Encouraging Insight

Adlerians focus on the here-and-now aspect of behaviors and on understanding the impact of one's expectations and anticipation on future events. These expectations can lead to faulty goals. Adlerians use therapeutic confrontation to help clients gain insight into these self-defeating behaviors and mistaken goals. Interpretations provided by the therapist not only encourage and challenge the client, but also allow for tentative hypotheses to be uncovered. Since Adlerians believe that no one can truly understand exactly what another is experiencing, they use questions and statements in order to present alternative theories. Open ended questions are used to help the client open up about thoughts and feelings. It is important that when the therapist provides the client with a hypothesis that is rejected, the therapist has the humility to accept that. This process is vital for client to understand their role in creating problems, how they are contributing to those situations, and how they can use possible solutions to correct those difficulties.

Phase Four: Techniques used in shifting a Client's Paradigm

The final objective in Adlerian counseling focuses on putting solutions into practice. This phase helps people find new and functional alternatives to behavior through acting "as if" they are the person they want to be. Techniques in this phase are designed to overcome feelings of inferiority and provide opportunities for growth. Therapists encourage clients to catch themselves in old patterns of behavior and use this insight to set new goals. By putting these new tasks into action, they are able to create change. This phase is important because it allows the client to solve problems, try alternative solutions, and identify which ones are the most important. Adlerians use a variety of experiential, cognitive, and behavioral techniques to help clients take risks and gain the courage to make changes. This approach is eclectic in nature. It is flexible, allowing the therapist to select techniques which are unique for each client. Some of the techniques used are as follows:

Push Button Technique: The Push Button Technique is designed to help a client identify their own role in creating and maintaining their own unpleasant feelings. There are three phases to the Push Button Technique (Mosak & Maniacci, 1998).

> Step 1: The therapist askes the client to close their eyes and recall a very pleasant memory. It must be pleasant enough to evoke positive emotions such as happiness or love. The client should recall the memory in as much detail as possible, then focus on the positive feelings that the memory generates.

> Step 2: The client is now asked to think about a memory which evokes negative or unpleasant emotions such as sadness, anger, or isolation. As before, the client should recall the memory in as much detail as possible, then focus on the negative feelings.

> Step 3: Client is either asked to generate a new happy memory, or to return to the one they used in step 1. Once again, they are asked to recall the memory in as much detail as possible, focusing on the emotion.

Once these three steps are completed, they are asked to open their eyes and share with the therapist what they have learned from this exercise. The hope is that the client has connected thoughts to feelings. If they have not, then it is the therapist's job to help them do so.
Once the connection has been made, the client is given Push Button Homework, and is asked to take two make-believe push buttons home, one negative and one positive. When they push the negative button, they are instructed to bring up an image or memory that has negative feelings associated with it, and vice versa. The client should then pick times throughout the week to use

these buttons. When they return for their next session, the therapist helps the client process what they have learned by helping the client determine which button they chose to push the most, and why.

The Question: During therapy the counselor typically utilizes a questioning technique in order to help the client determine the behaviors they would like to change. Different questions are utilized at different times during therapy. For example, a question during the early phases of therapy might be "since our last session, have you made any changes towards finding a solution to your problem?" A follow-up question could be "what behaviors do you need to change to get to that life?"

If sufficient progress is not occurring during therapy, additional questions may be asked to shed insight onto the problem. For example, the counselor could ask the client to describe how their life would be different if their problem magically disappeared.

Reflecting As If: Reflecting as if is an integrative and reflective process that can be utilized prior to the Acting As If technique. It is a method in which the therapist encourages the client to think about how they would be different if they were "acting as if" they were the person they want to be. The therapist might ask questions such as: how was your life different when you were doing this exercise? Did you learn anything from doing this assignment?

Acting As If: Once a client has thought about how their life would be different, the therapist might ask the client to Act "As If" they are the person they want to be until the next session. In this technique the counselor is asking the client to take a courageous step toward the life they desire. The therapist should have the expectation that the client can indeed follow through on this assignment. When the client returns for the next session, the therapist will have the client process how their life was, or was not different when they applied this technique. If the client successfully completes this task, it helps them understand that they must change their actions in order to elicit changes in their environment and social interactions.

Catching Oneself: In a therapy session, clients often identify a specific behavior they would like to change. Asking a client to catch oneself while they are engaged in the self-destructive behavior or irrational thought is one way the therapist is able to provide the client with skills to determine how to change this pattern. The goal is for the client to catch themselves without self-condemnation, take a deep breath, and change their behavior.

Spitting In The Soup: This technique is used to help a client become conscious of a manipulative behavior that they are unaware of or is inconsistent with conscious goals. Clients are often not cognizant that they are utilizing a behavior because of the pay off. For instance, a woman might say how ugly she is in order to get her spouse to tell her how beautiful she is. In this case the therapist would point out the manipulation. The hope is that by making the client aware of the behavior, they may no longer derive enjoyment from their manipulation.

Twelve Stages of Adlerian Therapy

Within the framework of the four phases or objectives utilized in Adlerian therapy, Henry T. Stein began to see a pattern emerge while analyzing the therapeutic techniques of Sophia de Vries. She had been practicing Adlerian Therapy with clients for more than 50 years and had studied under Alfred Adler. Stein (1988) studied their work and realized that 12 stages existed among the four phases. The twelve stages are as follows:

1) <u>Empathy and Relationship</u>
Because clients expect the therapist to "cure" them, the therapist must help the client to understand that in order to work together they must develop a collaborative relationship. Rapport is an important part of the initial stages of therapy. It is typically developed through the use of empathy, warmth, and acceptance. A therapeutic environment of hope, reassurance, and encouragement is needed for the client to desire the continuation of therapy.

2) <u>Information Stage</u>
This stage of therapy is intended to help the therapist gather relevant information about the client. Initially the client must be given time to talk freely, without structure. Eventually the therapist begins to gather information such as early childhood memories, family constellation, birth order, and reoccurring dreams. Information can be gathered through the use of a life style questionnaire, and from questions and active listening on the part of the therapist. During this stage of therapy, therapists provide their interpretation of behaviors that may be causing the client distress.

3) <u>Clarification Stage</u>
In this stage the therapist often utilizes Socratic questioning in order to help the client recognize their mistaken logic. Clients tend to blame others for their behavior, failing to take responsibility for their own actions. The goal in this stage is to help the client move toward more logical thinking, allowing them to accept responsibility.

4) <u>Encouragement Stage</u>
During this stage the client is encouraged to move away from old habits and behaviors. The therapist helps the client to recognize their accomplishments, and to do so humbly, not making too much of their progress. Strengths, assets, and accomplishments are recognized and facilitate the client's movement into the next stage.

5) <u>Interpretation and Recognition Stage</u>
During this stage of therapy, the therapist not only listens to the client, but also observes their behavior to determine if they match. In cases where words and actions do not match, it is the job of the therapist to confront the client and help illuminate the subconscious reason for their behavior. This is the stage in which the therapist presents their own interpretations of the client's behavior. This process helps the client recognize their faulty belief system. For example, if a client tells you she is not a type A personality, and she arrives 15 minutes early, and takes diligent notes that impact the effectiveness of the therapy session, the behavior contradicts the belief about herself. The therapist may even

know that the particular client got a 4.2 GPA in school. By using past and present behaviors, the therapist then challenges the client's belief about being a laid-back person.

6) Knowing Stage
   This is the stage in therapy where the client begins interpreting their own situations and then discusses them with the therapist. This allows the therapist to help them ensure that their own interpretation is logical. By doing so, the client recognizes their own personal logic that has been applied to their life, which has led to faulty beliefs. It is not uncommon in this stage for the client to believe that therapy is finished. It is the therapist's job to ensure that they stay engaged.

7) The Missing Experience Stage
   In cases where sustained change does not seem to occur, and emotional break throughs are far and few between, it is often necessary for the therapist to determine if the client has a missing developmental experience in their past. Reasons for missing development may include not feeling accepted by parents, feeling that all challenge in childhood were negative, or poor sibling attachment. For these clients it is important for the therapist to help the client gain these experiences through the use of guided imagery, role playing, or narration. This will help the client to make breakthroughs they were unable to obtain beforehand, and view their challenges in a more creative and healthy way.

8) Doing Differently
   In this stage the client must take their insights and put them into action. This helps the client to increase their confidence as they move forward, and assists in solidifying their new way of thinking. This can be done through small experimental steps. If the client is not moving forward with the new behavior, it may be necessary for the therapist to develop environmental strategies to help the client recognize that their old behavior will still lead to negative consequences.

9) Reinforcement Stage
   Encouragement is an important ingredient to facilitate the clients courageous move toward change. Because of this, the Reinforcement Stage is important to provide support for any change the client makes, whether through thought or behavior. Often times, the therapist will notice small changes before the client. This makes encouragement vital to the process. It helps the client notice what is or is not working. However, the therapist must be in tune with the client enough to recognize when encouragement will support positive change, and when it will prevent growth by giving the client a false perception of doing better than they really are.

10) Social Interest Stage
    According to Adler, psychotherapy is a practice and test of cooperation. This idea is central to the social interest stage. During this phase of therapy, the client moves from a self-centered position to one of being more outward focused. This allows the client to be

more cooperative with the therapist and with those around them and is important to the client, as it allows the client to participate in their personal relationships, as well as in community life.

11) <u>Goal Redirection Stage</u>
During this phase of therapy, the client should be letting go of their old perceptions of self, as well as their previous goals. The client is encouraged to develop new goals that are flexible and socially conscious. This allows the client see life from a healthier perspective. When this stage comes to completion, the client should be able to create effective goals, which in turn should provide the person with a more secure sense of self.

12) <u>Support and Launching Stage</u>
At this point in therapy the client has achieved self-worth and confidence. They have learned to enjoy challenges and growth in their life. They are now able to develop realistic goals for the future and have let go of old and rigid thinking. The client no longer perceives himself to be better or worse than other people in his or her community. At this point, some clients need an after-care plan as they leave therapy. This helps them to continue to challenge and develop their new self.

Examples of Therapeutic Sessions

The first thing that must be done in every session is to go over basic paperwork, which includes limits of confidentiality. This must be done before you get to know the person, regardless of what theoretical type of therapy you choose to practice. Find examples of paperwork, and how to have this discussion in the Appendix.

Adlerian's believe that the therapist and client are equals. The therapist does not want to put anything between himself and the client that would distract or separate himself, such as a desk.

Session 1: Empathy and Relationship Building

T – Hello Donny. How are you today?

D – Fine.

T – I thought we could spend a few minutes just getting to know each other. So, tell me a little bit about yourself. What are your hobbies?

Analysis: Each client has a subjective view of the world which the therapist must understand to facilitate change. Subjective lenses through which clients view the world include feelings, beliefs, values, and convictions. As humans, we use this information to come to certain conclusions about life. This information is used to understand a client's Lifestyle.

D – I like to do a lot of things. On the weekends we go dirt bike riding. I like to weld. My parents bought me the equipment.

T – What kind of things do you weld?

D – I like to take things like coffee cans and nails and turn them into various pieces of artwork.

T – That's amazing. Why do you like to weld?

D – When I weld, I am in a different world. There are no teachers to tell me I am doing it wrong. I am in charge. I can do what I want, be creative. There are no rules to follow, no spelling or math to get in the way. I can just be myself.

T – Do teachers tell you that you are doing things wrong often?

D – Yes, every day, every class. They make sure that I know I am stupid.

T – What does that look like?

> *Analysis:* Adlerian therapists guide the session through Socratic Questioning. The idea is that the client will eventually learn how to question their own mistaken goals and faulty assumptions.

D – Well, I have learning disabilities and most teachers don't really know what that means. To them, that means I can never really learn anything. I'm just kind of taking up space in the room. I'm at this private school, so I think that they don't always know how I got in or why I am there. I am pretty sure I am the first kid they have ever had with learning disabilities. My parents went to all these meetings to get me in.

T – So what do you think? Do you belong at the school? Or do you think your parents just pushed until they go their way?

D – No one really understands learning disabilities. The psychologists get it, but the teachers don't. So, no matter where I went to school, I think I would still feel this way. It's been like this my whole life. But this school teaches mechanics so I am really glad my parents worked so hard to get me in. I just wish they would pay more attention to what I can do. Then they would see that I'm not really stupid. It is just the world that thinks I am stupid.

> *Analysis:* As individuals, we each have a private logic that has developed in context to our experiences. When the private logic of a client does not match up to societal expectations, then problems arise. This leads a client to create basic mistakes within their private logic. Therapy focuses on helping the client identify and correct these basic

mistakes. Donny's private logic is beginning to surface in his comment that the world thinks he is stupid.

T – You keep talking about teachers making you feel stupid. Can you give me a specific example?

D – I did this one homework assignment; I got all the mechanics right. But because I didn't get the spelling right the teacher decided I was stupid and he failed me.

T – Can you explain that? What do you mean, you got all the mechanics right?

D – I knew exactly how to put the combustible engine together, but because I couldn't spell the words correctly on my report, I got an F.

T – I can see how that would be frustrating. Do you feel like you have had difficulty with teachers your entire life? Can you give me an example of the first time you remember having difficulty with a teacher?

> *Analysis:* Another technique utilized by Adlerians is early recollections. These memories are provided by the client in clear detail. Adler reasoned that out of the millions of memories, people remember one's that create our subjective world view and belief of self.

D – I remember this one time with my Kindergarten teacher. She wanted me to paint on this easel so I did. I took the brush and some black paint and started my painting. It wasn't good enough for her because I was painting in black. She insisted that I paint with color. I didn't want to add color to my painting. I liked the color black. She insisted it wasn't a color. I insisted it was. She yelled and tried to prove me wrong. Eventually I just threw the paint at her.

T – How were you feeling when you threw the paint at her?

D – She was frustrating me by being stupid. You don't ask a kid to paint and then tell them what colors to use. See what I mean? Teachers are always telling me that I'm wrong.

T – Wow! I can see how you have come to that conclusion. I think we are going to stop there for now. I have a questionnaire I would like you to complete for the next session. It will just give me a good idea about your childhood, your relationships with your various family members, and how you generally think about the world. It is my understanding that you have done psycho-analysis before.

D – Yes. But he never gave me a questionnaire to fill out.
T – (laughs). Probably not. Adlerian Therapy is a little different so I just want to give you a little information about it. Adlerians believes that people are creative, so you play a role in how you see the world. Some of what you believe about the world is pretty accurate. Some of it is more

just your own perception. You will talk about your past, but our goal is to figure out what is accurate, and what faulty or mistaken perceptions you have created. Are you up for it?

D – I'm not sure. That's allot of homework, and I already have enough. Can't we just talk about it? You probably won't be able to read what I write anyway.

T – Don't worry about spelling. Answers don't have to be in full sentences. There is no deadline for this. It will just help guide our sessions together. Do you think you can do that?

D – I can give it a try.

T – Great! I'll see you next week.

> *Analysis:* Donny believes that he can't do anything because he is dyslexic and he is projecting that belief onto everyone around him by stating that they all think he is stupid. Subsequently he is angry and does not communicate to the teachers what his academic needs are. Poor interpersonal relationships are products of misperceptions, inaccurate conclusions, and unwarranted anticipations incorporated into the lifestyle. Donny's hyperactivity probably affects him more than his dyslexia. He also believes he cannot become independent because of his disabilities.

Session 2: Information gathering stage

T – Welcome back! I hope you had a great week. I want to start our session by revisiting our discussion about your kindergarten teacher. We were talking about the difficulty she gave you about using black paint.

D – Why do we have to talk about this again?

T – Well by talking about early experiences, I am able to understand you better. I can start to see a connection between early experiences and your current difficulties. Does that make sense?

D – I guess so.

T – How about this, we don't have to talk about your kindergarten experience. Instead, why don't you tell me about your earliest childhood memory?

> *Analysis:* Adlerians typically ask for more than one early memory in order to understand where the client's perspective has come from. Above, it naturally flowed to ask about Donny's earliest school recollection. Now, the therapist is asking about the very first thing the client remembers.

D – Here is the sheet I filled out. It answers your question about that.

T – You did a good job filling out this form. I want to hear about your memories. Which one of these three memories is your earliest? What's up with that expression?

D – Are you kidding? What did I fill out the form for? My writing is horrible. You know I'm dyslexic right?

T – Well you completed everything I asked you to do and this is a hard form to fill out.

D – Thanks.

T – So let's get back to what we were discussing. Which memory would you say is your earliest?

> *Analysis:* Early childhood memories are important for Adlerian therapists because children form conclusions on the basis of subjective experiences. Because young children's logical processes are not highly developed, many of their conclusions contain errors and children accept these faulty conclusions as truths.

D – Ok, well we used to live near this family in Claremont. The guy was remodeling the house next door to ours. I liked to go over and play while he was doing that. When I got there, the first thing I would do was climb up the wall and through this hole into the attic crawl space. I loved the reaction that I got from this guy because I never used a ladder. My parents have always said that the wall was about 10 feet tall. One night, when the sun was going down, I ran over to check out what the guy was doing. I did my usual climb into the attic crawl space. I crawled over to the next room to check it out. I thought I was just jumping back down to the floor in the other room. Because there wasn't enough light in the room, I didn't see the hole in the ground. I fell directly through to the basement. It didn't really scare me, but it was really embarrassing so I didn't go back much after that.

> *Analysis:* By talking to Donny about his various childhood memories, we are trying to get an understanding of his subjective self-concept and self-ideal. Discrepancies between the two leads to feelings of inferiority. In this story it is noted that Donny has a low sense of fear, a high pain threshold, and is clearly an active child who does not like to be confined. By helping Donny correct false beliefs in future sessions, he can then see his life in a more accurate way.

T – Wow that's quite a story. How old do you think you were when this happened?

D – Probably around 3.

T – It's interesting, you mentioned this didn't scare you; that kind of surprises me.

D – Well, why would it scare me?

T – It would scare most children. Did it hurt?

D – No, not really.

T – Can you tell me about a time when you did get hurt?

D – Yeah. (small laugh). When we lived in Newton Highlands, Massachusetts, I use to ride my bike with my sister Susan and our friend Mark. We had this one ride out to Needham that we loved to take. We would ride out, get water at a local restaurant, and then play around on the nearby boulders. I remember this one time we sped off on our bikes as usual. We made it to the boulders and were playing around. Suddenly we heard our names being called. It was my mom. We were shocked because we didn't even think our parents knew where we were. They yelled up and told us to get home because the Donawicks had come into town with their plane and wanted to give us a ride. We jumped on our bikes and sped off down the hill. When I got to the bottom of the hill, my tires hit a pile of dirt and I slid across the sidewalk. I ended up falling off and Mark plowed into me. When I looked up, there were 4 adults standing around us. Of course, one of them was a nurse and I was so embarrassed. My sister ran across the street and called our parents from the gas station. They ended up having to take me to the hospital to get stitches in my knees. All I could think about while I was sitting in the ER was that I couldn't go on the plane ride.

> *Analysis:* Adlerian therapy is structured in a manner that helps the client understand that they are responsible for creating their own problems, faulty perceptions, and values. By helping the client learn to take responsibility for their own actions and behaviors that lead to the faulty thinking, the client can then begin to correct these issues.

T – That sounds painful.

D – It kind of was, but I was more upset about missing the ride.

T – Sorry you missed the plane ride.

D – Well we got to go the next day.

T – Did all three of you get to go?

D – I don't remember.

T – Is Mark a good friend of yours?

D – Yeah, he was when we lived in Boston.

T – How did you know him?

D – We knew him from school. We went to grade school together.

T – Were you in the same classes?

D – We were, but I only went to grade school for half a day when we lived there.

T – How is that possible? How were you able to go for half a day?

D – It was part of my IEP. I'm not very good at sitting still for a long time and I had a really difficult time doing classwork. So, the school decided that I would benefit more from only being in school for a half day.

T – Did you like this arrangement or did you feel like you were missing out on anything?

D – I really liked going for a half day. I remember that when I would go to school in California, before moving to Boston, I would give my mom a really hard time before school. I would kick, scream, cry, crawl under the bed, and generally do whatever I could to not go to school. From early on I knew that my teachers didn't think I was able to do anything academic; especially reading. I was never good at reading anything.

T – That's interesting. Did you hate school even when you were little, like pre-school age?

D – I don't ever remember liking school. I feel like I was always getting yelled at.

T – Were you getting yelled at by the teachers or by the students?

D – The teachers were the ones who were always yelling at me. I got along with other kids. The kids loved me because I would do things that they would be scared to try.

T – Like what?

D – I loved to climb curtains.

T – Well, now I know why you were getting yelled at. (Smiles). It sounds like you were quite an active child.

D – (Laughs). I guess I was a handful.
T – I enjoyed listening to you talk about your memories today. I would like you to think about school memories over the next week. Maybe write a few down; especially if they stand out. We will meet again next week, same time and place.

Session 3: Clarification

Analysis: In this session the therapist will utilize various types of Socratic Questions in order to clarify that the therapist understands the faulty beliefs that are hindering the client from moving forward. There are several types of Socratic Questions. This session will highlight a few of those.

T – Good to see you today. I thought we would take a few minutes and talk about some insights that came out of our last session.

D – We had insights?

T – Well, let's talk about them and see. I have a few ideas of my own. Why don't I share them and you can let me know if you think I am right.

D – That's fine.

T – Let's talk about school in Boston. You mentioned that you went to school half days because the teachers didn't think that you could handle more. How do you think school would have been different there, if the teachers believed that despite your learning disabilities you could indeed keep up with your classmates?

> *Analysis:* Here, the therapist is using a questioning style called Considering Alternatives. It helps the client think more logically about the issue being discussed. By thinking logically through a problem, clients may experience a paradigm shift that allows them to see the benefit of alternative behaviors.

D – But they didn't.

T – I understand that, but how do you think school would have been different for you if they did?

D – I probably would have failed out!

T – And you assume that because?

> *Analysis:* This is an Information Gathering Question. It is being utilized here to help the client be more concrete, as his thinking is vague and based on a faulty assumption. It is also being asked to help the therapist understand the client's subjective meaning.

D – Because I have learning disabilities!

T – Why does someone with learning disabilities have to fail out?

> *Analysis:* This question is called an Analysis Question. The therapist is asking the client for evidence to support the conclusion that he consistently makes, that because of his

learning disability he cannot succeed in education. It is forcing Donny to determine if his conclusion is actually logical.

D – Are you serious? It makes it harder for me to learn. I can't read as fast as other people, if, I can even read at all sometimes. How can I keep up with school?

T – How do you do with listening?

> *Analysis:* Here, the therapist uses another Information Gathering question to encourage a paradigm shift in Donny's thinking, and help him begin to determine the strengths he has to work through issues.

D – I am listening!

T – Yes. You are. But how do you think things would change if you had to listen to your text books instead of reading them? Do you think that you could gather the same information from the book that your peers do?

D – Oh. I never really thought about that. I have a great memory. Yeah, maybe.

T – So is learning the problem, or is reading the problem?

> *Analysis:* This is a Clarification Question. The therapist is trying to get Donny to change his definition of learning, so that he can begin to logically work through the weaknesses he has in obtaining information through reading.

D – Um, reading, I guess. I can learn things. I remember a lot. I am a great mechanic. I had to learn that. I just don't learn things the way the rest of my friends do. My teachers don't get that.

T – So, does that mean that if your teachers don't understand how you learn, then they automatically think that you are stupid?

D – Yes!

T – Do you think that you have the ability to help them understand otherwise? Are there things you can do to help them recognize that you are an intelligent young man who learns in a different way?

D – I'm sorry what? You want me to teach my teachers? How do you think they will do with that? They already think I'm stupid. You think they would listen to me, the difficult one? The one with the anger management issues? You do know that I have walked out of class before when they were pissing me off? I have no problem letting them know what I think of them.

T – So are they not giving you a chance, or are you not giving them a chance?

D – (Silence for a few minutes) I need to go away and think about that. That feels like an odd question. I don't know how to answer you.

T – That's OK. Our time is about up for today. I think this was a great session. Take time to think about that question this week, and then we can pick up here next week.

Session 4: Clarification, then move into Encouragement

T – Last week, I asked you if your teachers are not giving you a chance because of your disabilities? Or are you not giving them a chance because you assume they think you are stupid. Do you assume that they don't understand how to teach you?

> *Analysis:* Here the therapist is using a Clarification Question to determine if the paradigm shift has begun in the client since the last session. The goal here is to move Donny from feelings of inferiority based on faulty logic, to a place of logically evaluating his experiences.

D – Well, I guess that's valid. I think this one teacher really does think I am stupid. He barely looks at the content of the paper and really only grades me on my spelling. He fails me on almost all of my work, and it is going to cause me to fail out of this 5-year program I was trying to get through. If I go to my High School for 5 years, then I can get my High School Diploma and my AA Degree. But it is not like I have tried to sit down and talk to this guy. Not that I want to. He's a jerk.

T – I know you think he is a jerk, but what do you think would happen if you tried to sit down and talk to him?

> *Analysis:* Again, we are using a type of Socratic Questioning in order to get Donny to think about his problem logically and to identify alternatives. We are helping Donny move in a new direction by encouraging him to advocate for himself and individuate from his parents. By doing this we enter into the Encouragement Stage of therapy.

D – I don't think he would listen, he only listens to other adults.

T – That's interesting. So, what does that tell you?

D – What do you mean?

T – Well, you just stated that he listens to adults. So, what are your options?

D – I don't want to ask my parents to talk to my teacher.

T – Are they the only adults in your life?

D – Someone other than my parents? That would be great! They work and I hate making them take time off just so they can once again try to tell a teacher what to do.

T – Why not someone other than your parents? I know they probably understand your disability better than anyone else. But at some point, you need to be able to get support from other people too.

> *Analysis:* Because of Donny's disability he has over-relied on his family to provide for his needs. He is easily able to establish friendships, but unable to rely on them for support. The therapist is helping Donny with social interest by establishing a support system that extends beyond his family.

D – There is this one teacher that made me come talk to her after I turned in my first paper. She inked it up, but at the top of the paper she said "if this is a joke, come talk to me. If this is not a joke, come talk to me." She's been more helpful than most.

T – She sounds great! So, what is your next step?

D – I guess I need to talk to her and ask her if she would be willing to help me explain my disability to this guy.

T – You seem to be very knowledgeable about your disability and you are good at communication.

D – You mean talking? Haha.

T – Yes, you are very clear, and it's obvious that you are intelligent. Not many teenagers can express themselves like you do.

D – (smiles) So what do I do now?

T – So what do you think your next steps should be? You did the hard part, you identified someone that you feel comfortable talking to.

> *Analysis:* By asking questions that allow Donny to identify steps to change his environment, we are encouraging him to move beyond his faulty beliefs.

D – Well I have her class tomorrow. I'll ask her what she thinks about this idea. The worst she can say is no, right?

T – Right. Our time is up, but I am excited to hear how your discussion went next week.

Session 5: Interpretation and Recognition stage

T – Welcome back Donny. How did the conversation with your teacher go?

D – I did it. I talked to her and she said that she would go with me to talk with my shop teacher.

T – That's great! Did you talk to the shop teacher already?

D – This is the problem. She said that she would go with me; however, she wants me to set up the meeting with him.

T – That sounds fair. But I see from your expression that you don't like that option.

D – No. Did you forget that this guy doesn't like me?

T – I didn't forget that. But in the past, you said something about your parents talking to teachers. Were you not involved in those conversations?

D – They usually set up the meeting and I often go with them. But I'm there more to clarify what they are saying, like how much time it takes me to complete assignments, stuff like that. If someone were going to set up their own meeting it would be my sister Susan.

T – Oh, is she the oldest sibling?

D – No, why would you ask that?

> *Analysis:* The therapist is visiting birth order in this question to determine if Donny has any feelings of inferiority based on how each sibling behaves in the family system. Usually, the oldest child naturally takes on responsibility, as they are often helpful to parents when it comes to younger siblings. Also, because the older child often feels ousted by the next born, they take on responsibility to show their parents that they are superior to the younger sibling.

T – Siblings often take on certain roles based on their birth order. I know it is on your Lifestyle questionnaire, but just remind me of the birth order of you and your siblings.
D - I'm the oldest, Sue is two years younger than me, and Jo is 8 years younger than me. But Sue helps me with school work because she is good at it. She reads to me and corrects my papers for me sometimes.

T – So why do you think that your sister Susan would have the initiative to talk to her teachers?

D – Her teachers like her. She's a good student. She would probably just walk up to them before or after class and ask them if she could meet with them. She asks for tutoring sometimes.

> *Analysis:* Donny appears to simply give Susan credit for her educational abilities, but does not appear to feel inferior to her. His body language and chosen verbiage does not indicate sibling rivalry between the two.

T – So, if you acted as if you were Susan, how would you go about asking your teacher for a meeting? What would you say and when would you do it?

> *Analysis:* The therapist is asking Donny to utilize a technique called "Acting As If." The hope here is that by acting like his sister he will have the confidence to approach his teacher and ask for a meeting. Acting as if does not change the person instantaneously; however, it allows them to try a different role, and if they feel differently, then they will perhaps start to behave differently as well.

D – Actually, maybe I should go in at the beginning of the day, before classes get started. That way I can go into his office and ask him if he has time to meet with me. I'll let him know that my other teacher is coming with me too. That way he knows to set up a time when she can meet with us.

T – Great! So, what will you say? How you will you ask him for the meeting?

D – Let's see, I guess I would say "excuse me sir, can I talk to you for just a minute? I was hoping I could set up a meeting with you. Ms. Brown will be with me for the meeting. I just wanted to talk to you about a few things."

T – That sounds good! When are you going to do that?

D – Tomorrow, I guess.

T – So what are you going to do if you get nervous?

D – I don't know.

T- Why don't you try to act as if you are Susan?

D – (In a falsetto voice) Excuse me sir…

T – (Therapist laughs) You know what I mean. In your mind, when you enter the room, just act as if you are Susan asking for a meeting with your teacher. How does that sound.

D – Odd, but I'll give it a shot.

T – Can't wait to hear how it goes.

Session 6: Knowing

T – Hi Donny. How are you?

D – Good.

T – Did you get a chance to ask your teacher for a meeting?

D – Yes. We are meeting this Thursday. It was the only day that my two teacher's schedules lined up.

T – So, it sounds like it was a successful endeavor?

D – Yes. I did as you said. I acted like I was my sister and walked in with the idea in my head that he would just say yes because I am a good student and he likes me.

T – So why do you think your sister is so confident?

D – Well, she doesn't have learning disabilities. She cooks for us when mom is at work, she helps me with my homework. She did laundry while my mom was in the hospital. She functions more like the adult in the house then I do.

T – So wait, I'm sorry, was Susan born first? I thought you were.

D – I was. I'm the oldest child. She was the second born. Most of the time she acts like she is older though. When it comes to Jo, my youngest sister, I do act like her father sometimes, like when my parents go out to dinner, things like that.

> *Analysis:* Adlerians use five different labels for birth order: oldest child, second child middle child, youngest child, and only child. They recognize that some children fit into their role based on their birth order, but other times the way that they relate is not in line with when they were actually born. This can create awkward dynamics in the family. In Donny's case he is the first born, but it appears he functions like a middle child.

T – That's interesting. Listening to you, your sister acts like a first-born child. Does it bother you that she takes on more responsibility sometimes then you do? What is it like to have her help you with your homework?

D – Oh, I prefer it. It's much better. I'd way rather have my sister reading to me, then my mom or dad. I love them. They are great! But my sister and I are close, sometimes more like best friends. It can be a little hard on the self-esteem though. She is so much better at academics then I am.

> *Analysis:* Donny's perception that his younger sister is more advanced than he is academically can be a contributing factor to his lower self-esteem. This is where we see Donny exhibit some behaviors typical of a middle child.

T- So really, your mom, dad, and sister all advocate for you and take care of you. How could you take a more active role in your life?

D – It's not like I don't do anything for myself. I not only drive myself to school, but I drive other kids too. It helps pay for gas. I work at a gas station, although I do get help with writing sometimes. I do chores around the house. I build elaborate forts in the backyard. My mom and dad are really cool about that. I can cook a few things in the kitchen if I have too!

T – So you have all the skills to be independent. You work, you can make a few meals, you drive, obviously you dress yourself. You do chores around the house. So why do you feel like you are so dependent on so many people?

D – What do you mean? I have learning disabilities.

T – Yes. You do! What does that have to do with being independent?

D – What?

T – I think you should go home and think about it. In fact, try acting as if you are an independent adult this week. Then next week we can explore how that went for you.

> *Analysis:* For Donny, there is some perceived risk of being independent. He feels his learning disabilities preclude him growing up. The goal here is to get him to see that he is fully capable of being independent despite his learning disabilities.

Session 7: Emotional Breakthrough

T – Hi Donny. It is good to see you. How did your week go?

D – It actually went well. The meeting with my teacher went better than expected. He actually thanked me for coming in and said that he was proud of me for doing this without my parents. I didn't know what to say back. I really hadn't expected that reaction. It was really helpful to have Ms. Brown there, don't get me wrong, I still did most of the talking.

> *Analysis:* Donny is progressing through therapy and is beginning to acknowledge the difficulty that is contributing to his overall depressed symptoms. His faulty belief that his

learning disability is the reason why he couldn't become independent is starting to break down as he redefines what independence is.

T – So how did it feel to pretend you were an independent adult?

D – Kind of weird. I have really been afraid of getting out on my own. My parents have talked about buying me a mechanics shop, but my dad would have to do the books. That means that they would still be taking care of me. I wouldn't really be independent. So, I'm still struggling a little with the idea of being on my own. I'm not sure where my abilities to care for myself end, and where my parents need to always help begins. If they always have to help me, am I really independent?

T – (Chuckle) They are your parents. They are always going to be there to help you when you need it. It's in the job description. But I am curious, how do you define being independent? I am wondering if we have different definitions of that word.

D – Why? What's your definition?

> *Analysis:* The therapist is utilizing Socratic Questioning in order to break down faulty beliefs. Currently, Donny's notion of independence is unrealistic and causing anxiety and depression, as he does not feel that he is living up to those standards. As is typical with adolescent's, anger often masks internal feelings, and with Donny he is often frustrated and takes his anger out on his teachers. As Donny's definition of independence changes, his frustration tolerance should increase because he will have a more realistic view of what it looks like to function as an adult.

T – You first.

D – Being independent means that I can take care of everything myself, without any help from anyone else. I don't need dad to do the books at work. I don't need Sue to read to me. I can make it totally and completely on my own.

T – Interesting.

D – Why is that interesting?

T – I guess that I am not an independent adult then.

D – What do you mean?

T – Well, I am really bad at math, so I have hired someone to keep track of the books for me here at work. And I am really bad at house repairs so I have a handyman that does that for me.

D – Huh. Well, I guess that's true. I'm use to my parents doing everything themselves, from painting the house to putting up the wallpaper. They really don't hire people for much. Maybe they are a little different.

T – So, if your parents are different, and other people hire professionals to do that kind of work, what does that mean for you?

D – Maybe I really am more independent than I thought. I can open a shop, hire someone to do the books, and get on with life. Hey, I think we are done. Thanks doc.

T (Therapist laughs). We are certainly getting there, but we need to see you consistently act like an independent adult. What is something else that other people do for you?

> *Analysis:* Donny is struggling with the idea of his world view and there is discrepancy between his self-concept and self-ideal which contributes to inferiority.

D – Well, how do you get over the fact that when I was learning how to put an engine together, I read the book wrong and reversed the wiring? And I can't do the ordering because I tend to reverse the numbers.

T – OK, good point. What could you do?

D – Right now I work with one of my friends and he does the writing for me.

T – So how could you move to doing the writing for yourself.

D – Well, I could get them wrong. But that would probably get me fired.

T – Ok, let's pretend you own the shop. How could you make sure you got the order right?

D – Hire someone.

T – But if you had to do it, what would you do?

D – I guess my friend could look it over when I'm done.
T – That's perfect. So, if your friend checked it, does that violate your idea of being an independent adult?

D – Not by your definition.

T – And by yours?

D – I guess not. I've just always seen that as being dependent on others.

T – How do you define interdependence?

D – Inter what?

T – I am sure there are some things that your friend does not do well. Can you think of one? Are you able to do that well?

D – I'm a great mechanic. I could check his work under the hood, make sure everything got put back together correctly.

T – Do you understand interdependence now?

D – You each play to your strengths and help each other out?

T – That's right. Let's have you set a goal. What do you think of checking in with your friend and seeing if he is willing to check your receipts if you check his mechanical work? Can you do that?

> *Analysis:* Part of the difficulty Donny has is that his beliefs are based upon American values including independence. He believes that everything has to be done himself in order to be successful. The goal of the homework is for him to understand interdependence.

D – Sure.

T – Great! See you next week and I'll be excited to hear how goes.

Session 8: Doing Differently

T – Hi Donny. How are you doing?

D – Life sucks!

T – Not the answer I anticipated. Tell me why?

D – I got an F in that teacher's class. I went and talked to him, I thought he understood the problem, and he is still failing me.

> *Analysis:* This is a perfect example that therapy is not linear and patients can back slide.

T – So did you fail because of your spelling?

D – No! He didn't give us enough time to study. He knows it is hard for me to read and he gave us too much reading and a test the next day.

T – Do you have an IEP? Do you know what that is?

D – Yes, I've had an IEP forever. Don't you remember me telling you I was on half days before?

T – Are you aware of what is in your IEP? Your goals or accommodations?

D – Yes. Because I'm at a private school I don't have a special ed teacher. Instead, I have all these accommodations to help me. Like, I have 50% more time to read then other people do. I am supposed to be able to take untimed tests. I am supposed to be able to re-take tests that I fail.

T – So how do you use that information to advocate for yourself?

> *Analysis:* In the Doing Differently Stage, the therapist helps provide the client with insight through the use of concrete action-based changes. Therefore, asking Donny what he can do to advocate for himself allows him to identify a specific area where concrete changes can be made.

D – Argh. I don't like this adulting thing(laughs). I guess what you want me to say is that I'll go talk to him again, even though he should already know that I get to retake tests.

T – I understand your perspective. So how many students does your teacher see in a day?

> *Analysis:* Adlerians believe that no one can truly understand exactly what another person is experiencing, however they use questions and statements to present alternative theories. It is important for the client to begin to understand their role in creating problems.

D – Well, there are about 20 students in a class and about 6 classes a day; so, about 120 kids.

T – So how many of you are on an IEP?

D – Just me. Remember, my parents had to get me into this school because they don't have kids with learning disabilities. Oh, I wonder if he even knows what an IEP is?
T – He may not.

D – I guess I should go in and tell him that an accommodation on my IEP is the ability to retake tests that I fail. Then we can come up with a time for me to retake it.

T – I think that sounds like a plan. Now, I want to shift gears and talk about how you felt when you came in today.

D – I was pissed. Why?

T – We are going to try something. I want you to close your eyes and think of a very happy memory.

> *Analysis:* The therapist is going to use the push button technique. The therapist is using this technique here so that Donny can begin to gain control over his emotions. Without that control it is hard to assess the situation to determine if self-advocacy is appropriate.

D – Ok, I'm thinking about my first dirt bike.

T – Good. Now I want you to play the memory through in your mind, and then hold up a finger when you are finished. Think of it like a movie playing through your thoughts. Very funny Donnie, not that finger (laughs).

D – Ok. I'm done.

T – So how did you feel when watching that memory?

D – It was awesome. It was my first taste of independence. I got to test drive the bike, no one was in my ear telling me what to do. I was in charge. I can remember the smell of the bike shop where I got the dirt bike. It is a comforting smell for me.

T – Ok. That sounds great. So, what does happiness feel like inside?

D – It was a good memory. I feel calm. Everything feels lighter. My heart does not feel as heavy. I feel like I could smile.

T – Ok, now I would like for you to think of a memory of a time when you were really angry.

D – What do you mean? We just talked about that.

T – Let's pick a different memory.

D – Ok. Other than being angry with my teacher, I remember this one time when I had a bad fight with my parents. I was ready to stop going to school and they said I couldn't quit yet. They wanted me to finish the year out. I actually threw my brief case at my parents. I was pretty pissed.

T – Tell me how the anger makes you feel inside?

D – I feel like there is too much energy in my body. I want to run, fight, hit something. I need to release that energy.

T – Ok, now we need a happy memory. You can return to the one you just thought about or you can pick a new one.

D – I love it when we ride my bike with my cousins and hit the trails. This one time I rode the dirt bike with my mom on the back. I had so much fun spooking her. I would ride up to the edge of the cliff and she would scream "Donny, stop that!" It was hilarious.

T – That's good. Now you can open your eyes. How did that experience make you feel?

D – Well, why did you make me go from happy to angry to happy again. That didn't feel right. What do you want me to feel, angry or happy?

T – I want you to be connected to your feelings and realize how your body reacts. You can be in control of changing your emotions. Until you realize that you can control your emotions, you can get stuck in a single emotion. This happens more often with a negative emotion then a positive emotion. See how quickly you were able to go from happy to angry. You just said it yourself. You were happy, then angry, then happy again. That is all within your control. All you need to do is decide which button you want to push. To do that, we are actually going to practice.

D – Now?

T – No, you are going to do this at home. Here are two make-believe buttons. Your right thumb is your happy button and your left thumb is your angry or sad button. Over the next week, I want you to practice pushing these buttons and eliciting those memories.

D – Sounds like fun (sarcastic voice).

T – It will be (with extra enthusiasm). We will talk about it next week, and don't forget to talk to your teacher about retaking the test.

Session 9: Encouraging

T – So, how was your week?
D- Well, it wasn't the worst week ever. My teacher let me retake my test.

T – What did you get?

D – Well, since he didn't grade me on spelling, I got a B+.

T – What a difference that made, huh?

> *Analysis:* The therapist is encouraging Donny for a behavior he has followed through on. Therapists must be careful to encourage and not praise. Praise tells a child that you are

proud of them for conforming to a set of social rules set by you, the therapist, or by society. Encouragement, on the other hand, accepts the child where they are at. Encouragement statements identify effort on the part of the client. An example would be "I know advocating for yourself is hard for you, but look at the progress you have made and how that effort impacted your grade." Whereas praise would be "Wonderful job. I'm so proud of you." These two can be hard to separate out. This statement of praise, however, teaches dependence on the feedback of the therapist, instead of teaching the client to rely on internal validation.

D – Yeah, I guess it really did.

T – OK, well, let's talk about The Push Button exercise. Did you get a chance to practice it?

D – Sure.

T – OK, well, how many times did you practice it?

D – About 10. The world gives me some pretty good opportunities to do this.

T – What do you mean?

D – Well, when a teacher would piss me off, I would remember to practice. I did it when my parents made me mad too. It was great! I'd say, "wait, I need to go practice this thing to stop being mad. I'll be back." That pretty much diffused the whole thing. Thanks for that.

T – Well, you're welcome. Did you practice the button at all when you were happy?

D – What for?

T – To learn to get a grasp on the idea that you are in control of your emotions. You are supposed to practice the technique when nothing is happening. That way you can use it in the moment, so that you can deal with the issue instead of evading it by leaving the room.
Analysis: Instead of practicing the push button technique, Donny has used it to evade confrontation. The true purpose of the technique is to interrupt and shift from unpleasant and uncomfortable feelings to ones that engender more positive emotions. Clients often do not understand that feelings are a choice. Children and teenagers especially, look for external reasons for their feelings. That makes this technique crucial to working with Donny.

D – My parents harp on me too much. Sometimes I need an escape and you're a good excuse.

T – OK, so normally you practice the push button technique so you can learn how to gain control over your own emotions. Obviously, you used it when you were angry. How did that work?

D – When I was angry, I would hit it and I would feel better.

T – Did you think about your memory when you would hit your button? Or did the action of hitting it work for you?

D – Well the action of walking away from my parents worked.

T – I'm sure it did. That is more a time-out technique (small grin). It can also work to take a time-out. But we are working on the Push Button Technique. It will allow you to control your emotions more in-the-moment. What I would like you to do is to practice the technique when nothing is going on. This will help you understand what you actually feel. What do you feel emotionally, physically… Then, when you are pissed off at a teacher you can bring up those happy thoughts and feelings to change the anger.

D – That takes time. I don't have time.

T – It seems like you had a pretty good week. So why are you so cantankerous all of a sudden?

D – Because my girlfriend rode out to my session with me today. She's pissed off because we are not spending enough time together so we were going to "enjoy" the ride in. But all she did was complain about it the whole time. And then, because people know I am a mechanic, they've started dropping by to see if I can take a look at their car. I feel like I have to say yes. They are my friends. But I need to get my homework done. It is also hard to say no to them because since we go to different schools, I don't get to see them much anymore. See what I mean? I don't have time.

T – What a great way to give back to your community. You are mastering one of the 5 life tasks that lead to a more productive life. You are making a contribution to the larger world through your work, and helping others through friendship. So actually, you are mastering two. The five skills are: achieving intimacy, self-acceptance, developing your spiritual dimension, and the other two which you hit on, developing friends and work. When you mature in all 5 of these skills you should feel more confident in yourself, begin to see more success in advocating for yourself in the adult world, and you should feel more connected, which should help you feel less depressed. As far as not feeling so overwhelmed by lack of time, you may just need to put some boundaries on unexpected guests. Maybe people need set a time with you to look at their car. Or, maybe you can set a specific time during the week when they can drop by. This will allow you time to get your homework done, and to work on your Push Button Technique (big smile and slight chuckle).

D – Very funny (sarcastically). Obviously, this Push Button Technique is important to you.

T – Actually, no. It is important for you.

Analysis: The therapist is putting the responsibility back on Donny so that he will take ownership for the need to practice. The goal of Adlerian therapy is for the client to ultimately be able to make shifts and changes on their own.

D – Alright, alright, I'll practice it.

T – Great! That is the end of our session today. I look forward to hearing how your practicing went next week.

Summary of the Sessions

Although we hit on a number of important Adlerian topics and themes during these sessions with Donny, Adlerian therapy is not meant to be a brief therapeutic approach. Donny appears to be making progress towards alleviating some of his depressive symptoms. He still needs to develop the 5 skills necessary for social interest. In order to behave as a mature adult he needs to be able to advocate for himself and make healthy decisions. Currently, his decision are still based on false assumptions that stem from the low self-esteem he has developed due to the educational challenges that his learning disabilities have created for him.

He believes that he can not do anything because he is dyslexic. He is projecting that onto everyone around him by stating that they all think he is stupid. Subsequently he is angry that they think he is not intelligent so he does not communicate his academic needs to his teachers. Poor interpersonal relationships are products of misperceptions, inaccurate conclusions, and unwarranted anticipations incorporated in his lifestyle. Donny's hyperactivity probably affects him more than his dyslexia. He also believes he cannot become independent because of his dyslexia.

References

Adler, A. (1958). *The education of the individual*. Westport: Greenwood Publishing Group.

Adler, A. (2010). *Understanding human nature*. Mansfield Center: Martino Publishing.

Bottome, P. (1939). *Alfred Adler; A biography*. New York: G. P. Putnam.

Capuzzi, D., & Gross, D. R. (2007). *Counseling and psychotherapy: Theories and interventions* (4th ed.). New Jersey: Pearson Education Inc.

Corsini, R. J., & Wedding, D. (1995). *Current psychotherapies* (5th ed.). Itasca: F. E. Peacock Publishers Inc.

Corey, G. (1996). *Theory and practice of counseling and psychotherapy* (5th ed.). Pacific Grove: Brooks/Cole Publishing Company.

Kfir, N. (1991). *Personality & priorities: A typology*. Bloomington: AuthorHouse.

Mosak, H. H. (1995). Adlerian psychotherapy. In Corsini, R. J. & Wedding, D. (Eds.), *Current Psychotherapies* (5th ed.). Itasca: F. E. Peacock Publishers, Inc.

Mosak, H. H., & Maniacci, M. P. (1998). *Tactics in counseling and psychotherapy*. Brooks Cole.

Shulman, B. H. & Mosak, H. H. (1998). *Manual for life style assessment*. New York: Routledge.

Stein, H. T. (1988). Twelve stages of creative Adlerian psychotherapy. *Individual Psychology: Journal of Adlerian Theory, Research and Practice, 44*(2), 138-143.

SECTION IV: Existential Therapy

It is important to understand that Existential therapy has its roots in philosophy. Such philosophers as Soren Kierkegaard, Friedrich Nietzsche, and Jean-Paul Sartre had all identified themselves as Existential Philosophers. They understood well, our need to attribute greater meaning to experiences, and the need to identify to something greater than one's self. It was on the coat-tails of these philosophers that the following Psychologists found use for existential concepts in the therapeutic setting.

History of the founders

There are many founders of existential therapy. Viktor Frankl, Rollo May, and Irvin Yalom are often cited as the primary contributors.

Viktor Frankl. Viktor Frankl was born on March 26, 1905 in Vienna, Austria, and was reportedly close to his family. He was the middle of three children, born to a Jewish home. His father was employed as the Director of the Ministry of Social Services for the Austrian government. His mother was described as kindhearted and pious (Frankl, 2000).

Viktor was a thoughtful and inquisitive young child, often questioning life's nuances. At the age of three he decided to become a physician. By four, he was questioning the transitory nature of life and how death makes life meaningful (Frankl, 2000). Viktor was a very good student during his early educational career; however, during junior high he started spending more time researching areas of personal interest. This led to taking adult educational classes in Psychology during high school and a blossoming friendship with Sigmund Freud. Viktor sent Freud information that he "thought would interest" him (Frankl, 2000, p. 48) and Freud answered each correspondence.

Then, at the young age of 15, Viktor gave his first lecture. His talk was on "The Meaning of Life" (Vesely, 2020). Upon graduation from high school, he entered medical school at the University of Vienna, where he received both his MD and PhD. He studied both Neurology and Psychiatry, and specialized in depression and suicidality. While still in medical school he noticed that high school students seemed to commit suicide during finals. He started centers at high school campuses to counsel students during this time.

In 1942, he, his wife, children, and his parents were all captured and sent to Theresienstadt Concentration camp. Viktor was sent to four different concentration camps over a period of four years, and was finally liberated in 1945. It was at that time that he learned of the deaths of all his family, with the exception of his sister, who now lived in Australia (Frankl, 2000).

Frankle emerged from the war with the belief that no matter how much control a person had over you, they could not control your thoughts. One could still maintain their spiritual freedom within themselves, regardless of what was going on externally. This belief fueled his work with liberated victims of concentration camps, trying to address their depression and prevent suicide attempts. It was during this time that his logotherapy developed, helping the victims find meaning in their experiences during the war, as well as supporting their personal search for meaning (Frankl, 2000). Logotherapy became his primary contribution to existential therapy.

Irvin Yalom. Irvin Yalom was born in Washington, DC to Russian immigrant parents on June 13, 1931. His father owned a grocery store in a low-income neighborhood of segregated Washington, DC. The family lived in the second-floor apartment above the store. Living in a dangerous neighborhood afforded Irvin ample time indoors, reading. This pass time served a dual purpose. It kept him away from the violence, theft, and racial skirmishes that plagued his neighborhood, and also gave his parents the "satisfaction of knowing that they had begotten a scholar" (Yalom, 2017, p. 24). Irvin preferred reading at the Washington Central Library to reading at home. Not only did Irvin often feel out of place in the world, being the only white kid in a black neighborhood and the only Jew in a Christian world (Yalom, 2017), but he also did not have a good relationship with his mother. She was not one to speaking kindly to Irvin and tended to view him as unruly, disrespectful, and disruptive. In fact, at the age of 14, when his dad was having chest pains, and appeared close to death, his mother said to Irvin "you - you killed him." (Yalom, 2017, p. 12). Following this incident, Irvin made a conscious decision to stop interacting with his mother and they lived like strangers in the same house. Additionally, he felt disappointment towards his father for failing to stand up to his mother and support him. Around that time, while his older sister Jean was off at college, his family moved to a new house a block from Rock Creek Park. It was much larger than their apartment above the grocery store and offered an idyllic setting free of the filth, danger, and anti-Semitism that he was used to.

Upon graduating from high school, Irvin earned a full-tuition scholarship to attend George Washington University in Washington, DC; a fifteen-minute commute from his home. While Irvin had known that he wanted to be a doctor since the age of 14, when his father had a heart attack, he was aware that he had to overcome overwhelming odds, given that most medical schools had a strict 5 percent quota for Jewish students. This realization gave Irvin the drive to work hard and he obtained a straight A+ record in college. He applied to 19 medical schools and received 18 rejections and one acceptance to George Washington (GW) Medical School. Following his first year of medical school at GW, he decided to transfer to Boston University Medical School to be close to Marilyn, his future wife. They married on June 27, 1954. Irvin received his medical degree with a focus in Psychiatry.

After graduation from medical school, he entered into a one-year internship at Mount Sinai Hospital in New York, diagnosing and caring for patients. He rotated through several services during the year at Mount Sinai. Although no formal psychiatric rotation was offered, Irvin hung around the psychiatry department and attended numerous clinical and research presentations. After his time at Mount Sinai, Irvin entered into a psychiatric residency at John Hopkins in Baltimore. Following his three-year residency, Irvin was inducted into the army for two years of mandatory service. He was required to report for service at Tripler Hospital in Honolulu, Hawaii, and described his army duty as undemanding. He spent a majority of his time in an inpatient unit with most patients pretending to be mentally ill in order to be discharged. Following his time in Hawaii, they moved to California where Irvin began working at the Stanford Psychiatry

Department in Palo Alto. During this time, he wrote the "the first comprehensive textbook in existential psychiatry," (Corsini & Wedding, 1995) called Existential Psychotherapy.

For the next 15 years at Stanford, Irvin was heavily involved in group therapy where he employed existential therapy in a group setting. He also developed a strong connection to the Mental Research Institute (MRI) and "for an entire year I spent every Friday in an all-day conjoint family therapy course taught by Virginia Satir" (Yalon, 2017, p. 134). In 1967, Irvin received a career teaching award that allowed him to spend a year at the Tavistock Clinic in London. While in London, he was devoted to writing a group therapy textbook.

Rollo May. Rollo May was born on April 21, 1909 in Ada, Ohio. Although born in Ohio, he spent much of his childhood in Michigan. May's parents divorced when he was young. He was the oldest of six children and had a sister who was diagnosed with Schizophrenia. His mother would often leave the children alone in the home, which left May responsible for their care. This often-posed challenges for him (Pace, 1994).

When Rollo was old enough to attend college, he began his education at Michigan State University, in pursuit of a Bachelor of English. Within a short period of time, his involvement in a radical school magazine got him kicked out. May then decided to finish his degree at Oberlin College in Ohio.

After graduating with his BA in English, Rollo May headed to Europe where he traveled and taught at Anatolia College in Pilea Greece. While in Europe, he met and studied under Alfred Adler. Upon returning to the states, he worked as a counselor at Michigan State University for a short period, before moving to Manhattan to study Theology at Union Theological Seminary. Upon graduating from the Seminary, he served as Congregational Minister. He soon resigned to pursue a Doctorate of Psychology at Teachers College at Columbia University. During his study he contracted Tuberculosis and recovered in a sanitarium where he spent his time studying the works of Kierkegaard and other European Philosophers (Rollo May, 2015). During this time, he began to believe that humans could only be understood from a subjective point of view. He believed that anxiety in a human being created the need to search for the self, and felt that freedom, choice, and responsibility played a role in helping us determine our values and resolve our anxiety.

May was an extremely accomplished person. In 1939 he published the very first text on counseling in the United States, called the *Art of Counseling*. He went on to publish a total of 15 books. Not only was Rollo May known as one of the first to bring Existentialism to the United States, but he is also known for being one of the originators of the Humanistic Movement in Psychotherapy. He was the first to break from Freud's concept of Personality, and to stress that most of the human struggle emanated from anxiety. He was the founder of Saybrook Graduate School, and the co-founder of the Association of Humanistic Psychology. He passed away in San Francisco in 1994 (Pace, 1994).

Approaches to Existentialism

Existentialism often represents different perspectives and approaches (Capuzzi & Gross, 2007). For instance, you will hear people refer to dynamic and humanistic existentialists; both of whom focus on different aspects of existential theory. Dynamic existentialists are concerned with helping clients resolve inner conflicts and anxiety. Humanistic existentialists look at the whole person and that individual's unique experience. The notion of unconditional acceptance and authenticity play a key role during therapy.

Regardless of the perspective that the therapist comes from, all existential therapists are looking to help their patients understand and deal with their existential dilemma. This dilemma makes us aware of the fact that we are finite beings, without any specific quantified structure in life. We must utilize our own creativity to create this construct, in order to live a full, happy, and moral life in the world with which we find ourselves.

Major Constructs

Logotherapy is considered the "Third Viennese School of Psychotherapy," (Frankl, 2000, p. 30) following its predecessors; Freudian psychotherapy and Adler's individual psychology. The premise of logotherapy is to encourage the client to find meaning in their life and in life's circumstances; especially in circumstances when suffering was an integral part of the experience. Logotherapy challenges the client to confront their personal meaning in life and reorient their personal paradigm. When the client becomes aware of this meaning, they often find that they have the ability to overcome neurosis. This search for meaning is the primary motivation.

Viktor Frankl (Frankl, 1992) identified three main problems that man has to solve in order to identify meaning in life.

1. "The Essence of Existence." To determine the essence of existence, the client must figure out what he is responsible for and who he sees himself as being responsible to. The therapist will not allow the client to pass the responsibility of judgment to the therapist because meaning is individual to each person. The patient must decide if a task represents responsibility to society or to his own conscious.

2. "The Meaning of Love." To become aware of another human beings' experience, one must love that person. This type of love is interpreted as any intimate relationship driven not by sexual desires, but relationships. For example, the love between a parent and child, or between siblings, constitutes the love described by Frankl.

3. "The Meaning of Suffering." Human beings are often confronted with what they perceive as hopeless situations that cannot be changed. When indeed a situation cannot be changed, the human being is challenged to change their perception of their suffering. Frankl indicates that a client can find meaning in the midst of suffering.

Frankl's main way of interacting with clients was through Logotherapy, which utilizes 3 primary techniques.

Paradoxical intention is a technique that has the client focus on what is most feared. For example, if a client is scared of talking to strangers, the therapist would have him purposefully engage others in a dialogue during a social function.

De-reflection is a technique used when someone is overfocused in therapy on either themselves (self-absorption), an issue, or the attainment of a goal. When this happens during Logotherapy, the therapist will refocus the client away from self, in order to think about others, and the impact that they, the issue, or the goal may be having on others. This other focus helps them to live a more rounded and whole life, by encouraging them to see the whole world around them, instead of just considering themselves.

The technique of Socratic Dialogue requires that a therapist listen with total focus to the client as they describe their concern. The therapist can then point out the use of certain words or phrases, allowing the client to see new meaning in them. This particular technique is used to empower the client by helping them realize that the answers they are seeking are contained within (Logotherapy, 2015).

Whereas Frankl created a specific therapy model to interact with and guide clients through Existential Therapy, Irvin Yalom's approach to existential therapy focuses on "4 ultimate concerns" (Wedding & Corsini, 2019, p. 274).

1. Death: Existential anxiety exists within our awareness of death and the simultaneous need to live. He contends that this begins as a very young child and in order to cope with the terror of this realization we erect defense mechanisms to mask our awareness of inevitable death.

2. Freedom: Existential freedom refers to the notion that an individual is responsible for his or her actions. How much responsibility the individual is willing to accept for his or her life situation is directly related to how much anxiety they experience. If they see someone else as responsible for what happens in their life then the amount of anxiety will be higher than if the individual realizes that he or she is responsible to choose. Willingness is the ability of the individual to follow through and make change in their life. People tend to play the wish game (e.g., I wish my I had become a vet). You have to go from wishing to willing. People can be impulsive or compulsive (i.e., don't act). Once an individual experiences a wish (I wish I had become a vet) he or she is faced with a decision (to go back to school, or to continue with the current career). At times the individual may attempt to delegate (I already have a family; I can't go back to school) instead of attempting to make a decision on their own.

3. Isolation: This is related to the notion that we enter the world alone and exit the world alone. Therefore, no matter how often we are around others, we cannot fully share our consciousness with them. Many attempt to resolve their feelings of isolation with fusion. When a person fuses with another, they give up their own desires for that of the other, so that instead of living with "I," they can become a part of "we." Fusion underlies the idea of love and saves one from the isolation of being lonely.

4. Meaning: Individuals require meaning in their life that can be constructed by the individual to create a set of rules for which we live. From this schema we develop a hierarchy of values and how to live life.

Rollo May, also believed in four components to existential therapy. But because he focused on normal and neurotic anxiety, his fourth component was called meaninglessness. This alluded to the fact that people had to contend with the anxiety of having to create their own meaning, which contributed to the development of their personality.

May believed that neurotic anxiety was grounded in the early relationship between infants and their parents. For May, almost every crisis in a human being's life arises because of underlying anxiety. Some people perceive challenges as opportunities, while others perceive them as threats. In order for a client to understand their own anxiety, they need to understand it in relation to freedom. He also postulated that culture could affect a person's anxiety.

May believed that people lived a life long process called integration. In order to do that we have to separate ourself from the herd mentality and live a conscious, free, and responsible life. Because a person integrates throughout their life, a mature 9-year-old may be determining what qualities lead to a healthy friendship, whereas a healthy 20-year-old may be determining a career choice different from what friends or parents expected of them. The goal is for a person to make choices based upon their authentic selves and not based upon who others expect them to be. He proposed that for people who are able to do this, they would be able to experience joy and gratification.

May recognized that love was not just between mature adults. Instead, he spoke of 4 types of love that existed in Western Society. He called those 4 types of love: sex, eros, philia, and agape. He believed that to be a true mature adult, one must be capable of giving and receiving mature love.

Existential Concepts

Existential Crisis: How to lead a productive adult life. What am I going to do with my life?

The "I-Am" Experience: We conceptualize ourselves by status and profession, but that's not who we are. We are human beings living a life. Until we understand that it is us making decisions and not things being thrust upon us, we cannot make change. Therefore, the "I-Am" experience is the "science being" (Corsini & Wedding, 2005, p.270). It is common during the journey of self-realization for clients to explore the paradox of non-being.

Three Facets of the World: While there is an objective world that is made up of the environment, space, and time; we cannot discount our subjective experiences that impact how we make our choices. In existential therapy the Eigenwelt "own-world," is one's subjective experience (e.g., For me, that person is attractive). Umwelt "world around," encompasses the biological world (i.e., the need to eat, sleep, etc). Mitwelt "with-world," is us in relation to others (i.e., social environment, cultural environment). The Mitwelt and Umwelt blend together and facilitate the development of Eigenwelt. In other words, attraction is determined not only by biology but also from what society and culture deem to be attractive.

The Concept of Time: There are three facets of time, the actual clock (i.e., where 60 minutes make up an hour), the subjective experience of time (i.e., where an hour can seem like forever or only a minute), and the awareness of time (i.e., we aren't going to live forever and what are we going to do with that time). These three concepts impact the view of our experiences. Grief is a good example of the three experiences of time. It is common, during grief, to experience five minutes on the clock as three hours from a subjective experience. It is also common, to become aware that time on Earth is limited; which can launch the person into determining how they want to impact the world with the time they have left.

The Concept of Transcending Situations: Humans have the cognitive ability to transcend time and place. A person can think back to a bad incident and be limited by it or can see it as an opportunity to learn. Looking at the past, present, and future allows us to transcend the actual time we are in.

Concept of Therapy

Existential Therapy is unique in that there is no single founder. During Post WWII, many people in Europe began to question the existence of God. They had been placed in a situation where their mortality had been brought to the forefront of their mind. In struggling with this concept, Existential Therapy began to emerge all over Europe.

Early writers took note of the isolation created from broken families, families trying to reunite with their family members lost during the war, and the death of family members in concentration camps. This led to a desire to find meaning in their experiences.

The founders focused on the following propositions: the capacity for self-awareness, freedom and responsibility, striving for identity and relationship with others, the experience of aloneness, the search for meaning, anxiety as a condition for living, and awareness of death and non-being (Corey, 2019).

1. The ability to become self-aware: As humans, we have the capacity to become self-aware. Awareness and the decision to expand is fundamental to human growth. With growth, humans begin to understand that they are finite, we chose our actions and can partially create our own destiny, we realize that we can make new decisions and can chose how we react to those events.

2. The impact of freedom and responsibility: People are free to choose, which helps to create our own destinies and our own problems. Therefore, we have to accept the responsibility to guide our lives. People can choose not to do this by blaming external forces. Existential guilt is being aware of "choosing not to choose." Sartre said that "we are our choices." The therapist's role in this proposition is to help the client understand choices and consequences.

3. Developing identity and relationships with others: People are concerned with preserving their own uniqueness, but also with wanting to be able to relate to others. There are 4 stages of striving for identity and having relationships with other people: a) It takes courage to be who you are; b) the experience of being alone; c) the experience of relatedness; d) struggling with our identity:

    a. Courage to be who you are: It's easy in a relationship to take on someone else's values. Therefore, you must have the courage to be yourself. This requires identifying who you really are through questioning, creativity, and the understanding of your core being.

    b. The experience of being alone: By learning how to be alone we derive strength from within ourselves. This allows us to ascertain the meaning of life as an independent person. It also allows for self-discovery of our own strengths and weaknesses so that when we interact with others, we are enriched by their company, and they are enriched by ours.

    c. Understanding our need for affiliations: Relationships with others are important. We want to feel important to individuals and we want them to be important to us. When one has become comfortable being alone, the relationships that they seek are healthy and based on mutual fulfilment. If we are not comfortable being alone, then our relationships are often unhealthy.

    d. Seeking our own identity: because we are afraid of dealing with aloneness, people can get stuck in a state of doing, instead of just being. When we get stuck in a pattern of doing, we often engage in ritualistic type behaviors that we acquired in early childhood to reduce the anxiety of isolation.

4. The search for meaning: Humans struggle to develop a sense of purpose and wonder about how they will impact the world and what type of legacy they will leave behind. There are 3 stages:

    a. The void of discarding old values: Values guide our life decisions. As a child, we take on values from our parents; this may not work for us as we transition into adulthood. During therapy, clients may discard old values without having a new belief to replace it with. When a client begins to discard old values, it is the therapist's job to help the client learn to trust themselves to create new values that are more authentic. During this time of discovery, the client may feel unsettled with the lack of values to make decisions with.

    b. Living without meaning: Client's may feel like life is meaningless. Given the fact of our mortality, people may wonder why continue? Meaninglessness in life leads to emptiness. The feeling of meaninglessness is also known as *Existential neurosis*. Because there is no preordained way to live, clients need to develop their own meaning. *Existential guilt* grows out of incompleteness and guilt that the client has not lived up to their potential. If a person cannot solve the problem of creating meaning for themselves, they will feel empty and hollow. This experience is called the *Existential vacuum*. If someone becomes trapped by their feelings of emptiness, they may withdraw from trying to create purpose in their life.

    c. Developing new meaning: unlike the pessimistic view of existential philosophy, existential therapists believe that one can find meaning in their suffering. Suffering can be turned into human achievement if the individual allows for it. Logotherapy focuses on this premises. The therapist does not provide the meaning for the client, but helps them find meaning in their suffering and despair, and the client can ultimately triumph from the experience.

5. Anxiety as a part of daily life: Existential therapists have a broad definition of anxiety. They feel that anxiety is a part of daily living. It arises from our need to survive and persevere. This kind of normal anxiety, known as existential anxiety, can be a source of growth. Neurotic anxiety occurs when, for a client, it becomes disproportionate to their situation. It can paralyze an individual and prevent them from living in a productive way. A healthy life consists of learning to tolerate and become motivated by the normal anxiety in daily living. This can be done by taking a stance and confronting a dilemma. Anxiety becomes a mental illness when it becomes neurotic and debilitating.

6. Recognizing death and finality: Existential therapists do not view death as negative. Instead, awareness of death is viewed as part of the human condition that gives significance to life. Knowing that we do not have an eternity makes each moment in life vital. Developing an awareness of death can help clients to evaluate how they are living

and whether they are meeting their goals. Dealing with the inevitability of death helps us determine what accomplishments we want to make before we leave this Earth.

The Therapeutic Process

Existential Therapists emphasize our freedom to choose what to make of our circumstances. This approach is grounded in the idea that we are free and responsible for our choices and actions (Corey, 2019 p. 154). Although this is the framework that the therapist is working from, they do not guide what to talk about in the session. Instead, they look for opportunities to help the client find a clear view of their own life, within the framework of the tenants of existentialism.

The relationship between therapist and client is one of fellow travelers on a journey toward healthy interaction with life as it is now. Therapists focus on being empathetic with the client, to allow them to feel safe and confident in sharing information, and exploring their own responsibility and anxiety in reference to their current situation. In order to have this kind of relationship, the therapist must be transparent and vulnerable in the sessions, and should be willing to share their own life events, when appropriate.

Existential therapists are careful to live in the moment during the session, which is primarily guided by the client. The reason for this, is that the lack of structure within the session allows existential problems to arise naturally. By creating the therapeutic relationship, any tendencies that the client has in life, will come out in the session. For instance, if a client is controlling in their everyday life, then this behavior will also arise as the therapist and client journey together. The therapist can then point this behavior out to the client with such questions as, "I've noticed that there was some tension in the session today. You seemed to be focused on being in charge. Did you notice the same thing? How do you think that plays a role in your current life?" Because therapy is focused on road blocks in a person's life, therapists make sure they are not solving problems for the client, but eliciting the client to find solutions within themselves. The goal of existential therapy is to help the client learn how to solve their own existential issues in the future.

Existential therapists do ask questions revolving around dreams, as often times existential angst is being worked out in the mind during this time. Since the conscious mind is relaxed and non-judgmental while a person is asleep, much can be interpreted about dreams and their meaning in relation to therapy, as well as to the therapeutic relationship.

In essence, therapy is always creative and spontaneous. At the center of the session is a caring, human relationship between two people learning to manage the four concepts of existentialism: freedom, isolation, meaning of life, and death. Distinction does not exist between the client and the therapist because all people must manage and make meaning out of the four concepts discussed above.

Examples of Therapeutic Sessions

The first thing that must be done in the first session is to go over basic paperwork, which includes limits of confidentiality. This must be done before you get to know the person, regardless of what theoretical type of therapy you choose to practice. Find examples of paperwork, and how to have this discussion in the appendix.

Existential therapists believe that they are on equal footing with the client. While they don't discount the past, they typically encourage the client to stay in the present in order to live a better future. A patient may speak briefly about their past, but an existential therapist won't let them get stuck there.

Because existentialism is concerned with deep life changing questions, we are going to jump into session 2 where the client and therapist have already started to develop some rapport.
It is important to mention that this crisis was actually happening for this client in 1979-1980. So, going through this therapy session, we are going to stay in that time frame. Also, computers are a relatively new technology that were not yet available to the general public. So, there was some mild apprehension regarding how much they would take jobs away from the public. While they began putting computer technology into cars in the late 70's, this technology was only available in high end vehicles.

Session 2

T – Hi Donny. How are you?

D – I'm fine.

T – You don't sound fine.

D – Yeah, but that's what you want to hear isn't it?

T – Actually, I would rather you tell me how you are really feeling.

D – What do you want to hear about that for?

T – Existential therapy requires us to be open and honest for this to work.

D – Ok. You want to know the truth? I'm angry.

T – That's better. Why are you angry.

D – Because I'm going to have to live with my parents for the rest of my life. School's not going well, cars are changing. There is going to be nothing for me to do. Where do I fit in if I can't work? What am I supposed to do, flip burgers for the rest of my life?

T – What's wrong with flipping burgers?

D – Nothing! But I'm smarter than that.

T – Ok great! Then why don't you think your smart enough to do what you want to do in life?

> *Analysis*: This is the I-Am-Experience; Donny is struggling with the search for meaning. Six Propositions of existential experience. Donny is also experiencing meaninglessness (Yalom's 4 main existential concerns).

D – What do you know about fixing cars?

T – To be honest not a whole lot. Usually, I just take my car to a car expert, a mechanic.

D – (Smiling). I see what you're doing there.

T – chuckles.

D – So you know that mechanics do very hands-on work. It's just easy for me. I know what to do under the hood of a car. I get my hands dirty; I can see what's wrong with my eyes, I don't need some computer to tell me what's wrong.

T – How can a computer tell what's wrong with your car?

D – I don't know. Like right now, they are starting to put things in cars that you plug in and it tells you what's broken. It's only a matter of time before the computers are actually fixing the car.

T – Tell me your process for fixing cars?

D – Ok, well, first I talk with the owner of the car and they tell me what problems they are having. That helps me to determine what part of the car is broken. Then I pop the hood and see if the problem is obvious. If it is, then I fix the problem. If not, then I need to start to take pieces of the car apart to make sure that certain things aren't broken. Through a process of elimination, I am able to figure out what the problem is. I fix it. Then I call the owner of the car and tell them to pick it up.

T – Sounds like a good process. How could a computer detect a loose bolt making noise for the driver?

D – I don't know. I just know that computers seem to be taking over.

T – Ok. Let's talk about what can a computer do right now.

D – Well…they are mostly just reading numbers and processing data, I guess. I have actually seen a computer that takes up an entire room when I went to work with my dad.

T – Do you think that mechanic facilities would buy a computer that takes up an entire room?

D – Well when you put it that way, you're right. There wouldn't be anywhere to put the computer. But you know, they've shown us this video at school where computers are cooking and cleaning. They generally look like we do. That's more of what I'm afraid of. What if computers get so smart, they can open the hood of a car?

T – Well, I have a friend that programs computers. Don't people have to tell computers what to do and when? They don't have their own thought process.

D – But what if they do? What if that's our future?

> *Analysis*: Proposition of existential therapy: Anxiety as a part of daily life. Donny is currently experiencing neurotic anxiety, when a client's anxiety is disproportionate to their situation. It is the goal of the therapist to bring him around to existential or "normal" anxiety; which is part of daily life.

T – Ok, in this cartoon you're watching, what do the computers do?

D – They cook, they clean, and they talk to us just like humans.
T – Well at that point, is anyone going to be working?

D – You know doc, if that happens, you'd be in trouble too.

T – Well, I can always just do therapy with the robots. (Laughing). Ok, in all seriousness, I haven't seen the cartoon that you're talking about. But I have seen the Jetsons. In the Jetsons, they are driving around in flying cars, right? How far away from that do you think we are?

D – That's a bit far-fetched, don't you think? First off, I don't think we have the ability yet to put a jet engine in a car. And, most importantly, what would be the rules for driving? Does everyone get a pilot's license?

T - Good point. So aside from the rules and regulations of flying cars; how far away are we from having the mechanical parts available to create cars that fly? Is this a mechanical possibility at this time?

D – I don't know, you'd have to ask an airplane mechanic that question.

T- Ok, let's set that aside, and assume that right now it can't be done, or it would be. Now let's talk about computers thinking for themselves. Do you believe that we have the technology right now to make them do that?

D – I don't know, my friend at school made an R2D2 that could move around by itself.
T- Ok, so did it crash into anything?

D- No.

T- So how did it know not to crash into anything?

D – Well, it's like these little video cameras that sense it is too close to something.

T- Ok, but the computer did not think for itself, it utilized a sensor.

D – I get what you're saying. It didn't think for itself, it had sensors that helped it function.

T- So again, how long do you think it will be until computers think for themselves?

D- Well, we don't have that technology yet. Ok, problem solved, I'm fixed, no more therapy.

T- It's not that simple and there seem to be some other struggles that you are having. We'll talk next time.

Session 3

T – Hey Donny. Welcome back.

D – Hi

T – I've been reviewing my notes from your last session and I wanted to revisit a few things.

D – Oh great!

T – I wanted to talk a little about anxiety.

D – Ok, I know what anxiety is. I'm not sure why you want to talk about it though.

T – Tell me what it is.

D – Anxiety is for people who don't have any guts. They get all anxious about heights or getting hurt or falling off a motorcycle. They are afraid that if they go too fast, they'll get in a car accident. It's for people who really care about life.

T – It's for people who really care about life? What you do mean by that.

D – I'd rather go out Evil Knevil style, then get cancer and rot away.

T – Ok, well I can kind of understand that. But most people that feel that way, tend to go out Evil Knevil style when they get cancer. The way you phrased that, it's like you would be ok if you died tomorrow doing something reckless.

D – Reckless is the only time I feel alive. I don't even think of anything. I'm just in the moment. Analysis: While it does not appear that Donny is actually suicidal, it would be a good time for the therapist to do a suicide assessment to ascertain if he has a plan, means, method, or motive. It this session; however, we are going to continue forward as if the suicide assessment has already been conducted.

T – Just in the moment, let's talk about that phrase a little bit. Let's get a little deeper into how you feel when you are doing these things that other people consider reckless. You get this adrenaline rush that makes you feel more alive? You feel good like nothing can hurt you? What do you think about during those moments when you feel the adrenaline? Are you aware of what's around you? What's happening?

D – Ok, let's talk about when I climb up the chair lift at Mt. Baldy. I start to realize while I'm climbing, how far away the ground is, how small I am in comparison to the ground, how far away the mountains are, and how high they are. I start to realize that there are amazing things in this universe and my troubles go away for a little while.

T – So when you are doing that, it sounds like you are in the moment. In fact, you just described an existential moment.

D – What?

T – It is a moment when you are fully connected to the universe. You are looking in wonder at the things that are bigger and grander than you.

D – Bigger and grander than me, you mean like God?

> *Analysis*: In this moment, the therapist follows the client's lead in discussing their faith and religion. If you can't follow the client through their belief system then it is acceptable for the therapist to refer the client to another therapist.

T – Yes, God is bigger and grander than you. It sounds like, for you, these adrenalin rushes are a place of reflection and solitude with your creator. The adrenalin seems to focus you.

Analysis: Someone with ADHD may not necessarily respond to adrenalin in the same way as someone without it. In fact, they often create crisis to generate adrenalin to help foster engagement and focus in various situations.

D – So you're saying that an existential moment happens every time I get an adrenalin rush?

T – Maybe yes or maybe no. The existential moment is essentially when you realize how big the universe really is, and you are aware of the emptiness of life without values. During this time you feel awe and wonder and the pure emotional reaction to it. It's a special moment. Is this what happens each time you get an adrenalin rush?

D – No. Sometimes I'm just having fun and not really thinking about anything. Putting it in those terms, I think I've had one or two of those experiences; but they certainly do not happen every time.

T – Given what we were discussing, do you think you have an understanding of what an existential moment is?

D – Yeah, I think so. It's actually kind of interesting to learn about. I like this therapy much better than that Freudian stuff.

T – I'm so glad. I think we talked about a lot of deep stuff today. Why don't we call it quits and when you come back next week, we can talk more about how existentialism views anxiety.

Session 4

T – Welcome back Donny. How was your week?

D – It was ok. I had this test in my class. I was really worried about it because it wasn't just a technical test, which I would ace. It was a written exam and this guy grades me on my spelling. All my other teachers grade me on content.

T – How'd you do on the test? Did you get your results back?

D – Unfortunately, I failed; just like I thought. I swear this teacher is out to get me. It's just so frustrating.

T – Can you describe that feeling for me a little bit more.

D – What do you mean?

T – I'm talking about how you feel physically when you're frustrated.

D – Well, just before the test I get mad because this teacher is failing me just to fail me. It's hard to focus, I feel nauseous, my whole body has tension in it. I guess I would say that I'm anxious and angry.

T – Let's talk about the anxiety first and then we'll get to the anger. If you did not have dyslexia, do you think this would cause as much anxiety?

D – No, because then I could spell and I know this information forward and backward. But if I fail this class, I can't go into the 5-year program and I will never be able to move out of my parent's house. I will be dependent on them for the rest of my life.

T – I can remember when I felt that way. I was about your age. I was taking calculus. Because I have dyscalculia, I kept flipping numbers around and getting the wrong answer. I knew how to calculate the formulas. But when I would move the numbers over to a piece of paper, I'd put them in the wrong order. I needed this class to graduate from high school. I was so nervous that I would not graduate on time because of this.

D- What?

T – Yes. I do understand your struggle.

> *Analysis:* Existential therapists will share from their own life when appropriate to the session. This is part of being on the journey together. In this case, it has allowed the therapist to create greater rapport, by letting Donny know that the therapist has had similar struggles.

T - You were doing Freudian therapy before, correct?

D – Yes (eye roll).

T – Good. Well, Freudian therapists believe that anxiety is an unconscious worry, and that we will lose control of the id's urges. Did your previous therapist touch on what the id is?

D - Yes, we do not need to go there.

T – Perfect. Now, in existential therapy, the therapist believes that anxiety comes from one of 4 ultimate concerns: freedom, isolation, death, and meaninglessness. We don't have to hit on all those topics, but in your situation, I think it makes sense to talk about meaninglessness. Do you think this is affecting your life?

D – Well, if I fail this class and I can't get into the 5-year program, what am I going to do? I will have to live with my mom and dad. No one is going to marry the man who can't move out. What will I do to survive if I can't even buy my own food?

T- I hear what you're saying. That would concern me too if I were in your shoes. Now let's talk about how existentialists perceive anxiety. Anxiety is unavoidable. It is part of the human existence in this world. We need to learn to embrace it. By doing that, it opens us up to who we really are. So, let's get back to talking about your test. When did you first start worrying about it?

D- When I got the syllabus. I always look to see how many tests I have for the semester, especially with this teacher, because he's out to get me. I don't think he thinks I belong at this school.

T – So let me take a stab in the dark. Based on what you just said, do you think you belong at this school?

D – Well, I wouldn't have gotten in if my parents hadn't met with the administration. I'm the only person at the school with disabilities like mine. The other kids are academically inclined. I can see why my teacher might not think that I belong.

T – I understand that you have a specific set of learning issues, but everyone has something they have to deal with.

D – Mine are the most obvious on paper.

T – OK, so I understand that you may have the most trouble with paper exams, but if I understand correctly, you are brilliant when it comes to the actual mechanics of it. There could easily be kids who memorize answers well and spit them back on paper, but are struggling with the work under the hood of the car. Everyone has strengths and weaknesses, and your strengths are significant. You have an extremely high aptitude for mechanics. With that information, do you feel like you belong at Don Bosco?

D – Not really. I think this school focuses on academic achievement, even though they are teaching mechanics.

T – OK, where do you belong?

D – I don't know. I don't belong in regular school either.

T – What is a regular school?

D- You know, like Claremont High, the school in my town that all the kids go to. They are just as concerned with academics and they don't even have the mechanics program that Don Bosco does.

T – So, where is there a mechanics program that doesn't focus on academics?
D – There are some two-year programs, but you have to graduate from high school first.

T – We don't have much time left. I don't usually assign homework…

D – (Eye's roll)

T – but I would like you to take this week and explore what options you can pursue to become a mechanic. I am not sure that Don Bosco is the only way for you to do that. Does that sound good?

D – Actually, yeah, I think I can. See you next week doc.

Session 5

T – Hey Donny, how are you?

D – I'm pretty good, actually.

T – Oh yeah, tell me more?

D – I've really been thinking this through. I never really thought about other ways to become a mechanic. I was just so excited about the idea of the 5-year program at Don Bosco. But, after thinking about it, I think the GED makes more sense for me. I can even take it untimed. I can study for it on my own. While I am doing that, I can work for Dale, and learn mechanics and take the mechanics tests. I have already past the first one. That way, I can be earning money to move out of mom and dad's house, while I am working toward my GED.

T – That actually sounds like a great plan. It accomplishes more than one of your goals at the same time. Have you talked to your mom and dad about it yet?

D – Heck no!

T – Why not?

D – I think they still have their sights set on me completing at least a High School education.

T – Are you sure?

D – Well, they have worked really hard at helping me get through school.

T – But don't you think they would want you to be independent and happy?

D – Well, yeah, I'm just not sure they would see it that way.
T – Well, let's try something.

D – Uh oh!

T – Come on Donny, I haven't let you down yet. You think you can just try something for me? It's not homework. It's just a technique we use to help people work through future conversations. It's kind of like role playing, except you are going to face an empty chair and imagine that your parents are sitting in it.

D – Donny laughs

T – What's so funny?

D – Is my mom sitting on my dad's lap, or the other way around?

T – Therapist laughs. Who do you think it will be harder to talk to, your mom or your dad?

> *Analysis*: Existentialists often utilize role playing techniques as a means to help their clients process information. In this particular instance we are borrowing The Empty Chair Technique from Gestalt Therapy as a means of role playing for Donny. In the Empty Chair Technique, the therapist sets up a chair directly opposite the client. This allows the client to imagine the person they need to speak with is sitting across from them. The client proceeds to have the conversation. The client first sits in the seat of the client and begins the conversation. Then they sit in the empty chair and respond as they believe the other person will respond to them.

D- Let's start with my mom. I always hate letting her down. She has done so much to make sure that I received an education like everyone else.

T – OK. Perfect. I'm going to put this chair right across from you. I want you to face it and pretend that your mom is sitting in it. What would you say?

D – Hey mom. Any chance we can talk for a minute? (Donny turns to therapist) Now what?

T – Now I want you to get up and change chairs. When you sit in the other chair, I want you to pretend that you are your mother, and state what you think she would say.

D – (Looks sideways at therapist.) You're kidding, right?

T – Nope.

D- OK. (Gets up and slowly and sits down in the other chair.)

M - Sure. What do you want to talk about? (Donny looks at therapist.) Now do I move back?

T – Exactly. You are getting the hang of this.

D – Is this supposed to be a gym class, or a therapeutic technique?

T – Just hang in there with me.

D – Fine. Mom, I want to talk to you about school. (Donny changes chairs).

M – I know school has been rough. Just hang in there. We will get you more tutors and figure this out together.

> D – What if I don't want any more tutors?

> M – Well, what do you mean? How can we get you through Don Bosco, if we don't help you learn the material?

> D – What if there is another way for me to become a mechanic?

> M – Like what? (Sounding hesitant)

> D – What if I took the GED?

> M – I'm sorry, say that again?!

> D – What if I took the GED and went a different route to become a mechanic.

> M – I thought you wanted to get through the 5-year degree at Don Bosco so that you could have your Associates Degree. We have worked so hard to get you there.

> D – (Getting frustrated) It is becoming more clear each day, that is not going to happen. (Turns to the therapist) How much more of this do we have to do?

T – You are doing great! This is not an easy exercise. Think about a conversation you would have at dinner. What would that look like. How would your parent's talk to you?

D – Oh no! Here come the encyclopedias. (Donny laughs). Actually, I really enjoy dinner. Eventually someone brings up a subject and mom or dad tell us to go get the encyclopedias. Someone reads from it, usually my sister or my parents. They read better then Jo and I. They don't have disabilities. They get to be normal. Anyway, our dinner conversation revolves around the topic of the day, usually a question one of us has brought home from school.
T – That sounds fun. So, think about that kind of conversation. Close your eyes for a minute and tell me what you think your mom would say back to you if you brought this up at the dinner table, but it was only the two of you there.

M – (Donny moves to the empty chair) I can meet with administration and see what we can do about that. You're really only having trouble with one of the teachers, right? Maybe someone needs to sit him down and help him understand your disabilities.

D – I'm tired of the fight mom. There is more than one way for me to pursue my career. I could graduate from the high school program at Don Bosco and then go to a technical school, or I could take the GED, study under Dale, which I am already doing, and take my mechanics tests that way. I've really thought about all the options. School just keeps getting harder and harder. I think that I could study and work at the same time. Then I could move out in a year or two. What do you think?

M – I think we should talk to your dad about it. It sounds like you have really thought this through, and it sounds like you know what you want. I just don't want you giving up your dream because you think that you have to. But if it is what you really want, then it does sound like we could make that work. Have you talked to Dale about it yet?

D – Yeah! He said that if it was OK with you, he was willing to be my mentor and help me learn everything that I need to know to be a mechanic.

M – OK. Let's set a time to talk to dad, maybe this weekend. How does that sound?

D – Good. Do you think he will be mad?

M – No. He will just want to walk through it in a logical manner and make sure that it makes sense for you and that you can reach your goal that way. He just wants you to be able to be independent, and he wants you to be happy.

D – But you both have put so much time and effort and money into my education. Won't he be mad that I wasted that?

M – We did this so that you could live the life that you wanted. You are so intelligent Donny. We wanted you to have the same opportunities as everyone else. But if this gets you where you really want to go, he won't be mad. Nothing we have done for your education has been a waste.

D – Thanks mom. (Donny looks at the therapist) Am I done now?

T – How do you feel?

D – I feel stupid talking to an empty chair.

T – Is this where you expected this conversation to go?

D – No. I think after talking it through with an empty chair, that maybe they will be more accepting of this then I originally thought. I didn't even know how to start the conversation. At least I have an idea about how to do that now.

T – On a scale of 1-10 how much anxiety do you have about talking to your mom and dad now?

D – I am still pretty nervous, maybe a 6 or 7? But, at least now I know how I want to start the conversation, and I like the idea of going to one parent and talking it through, then getting help going to the other parent.

T – So do you feel like you can go through with this conversation before our next session?

D – (Deep breath) Yes. It will be hard, but yes.

T – Great. I'm looking forward to hearing how it went next week.

Session 6

T – Hi Donny, how was your week? Did you get a chance to speak with your parents?

D – My week was pretty good. I did talk to my mom and dad about changing directions with my approach to getting my mechanic's license.

T – So how did it go?

D – Pretty good. They want us to meet with the administration at Don Bosco one more time before I withdraw. (Donny looking in his lap as he answers).

T – How do you feel about that?

D – Well, it's a pain. I was hoping they would just let me withdraw. But they feel like I should talk to them about why I have made this decision.

T – Do you think that there is any value in that?

D – Well, I think that it will make my parents happy.

T – Anything else?

D – What do you mean? Is this about advocating for myself or something?

T – When I make a big life decision, I like to have closure so that I don't spend the rest of my life wondering if I made the right decision. So that is one thing that you can get out of the conversation. Don Bosco may need to hear you tell them why this isn't working. Your parents may need closure. There is allot of value that could come from having this conversation. But I really want to know if you think it has any kind of value.

D - Yes. I get to stop worrying about school, and start studying for my GED. I can just get on with my life when this conversation is finished.

T – It sounds like you are comfortable with this decision. One last thing that I would like to talk about, is that pretty early on in therapy we found that much of your anxiety was rooted in meaninglessness. How do you feel you have progressed with that?

D – I actually feel hopeful. I have always wanted to be a mechanic, and now I have a path forward. I have also worried about living with my parents for the rest of my life. But if I can earn a living while I am getting my GED, then that is a moot point.

T – So it seems like we have journeyed through much of what was blocking your way to becoming a successful mechanic. Let's just check back in a month and see how you are doing.

D – Great!

T – OK, so I will see you in a month.

References

Capuzzi, D., & Gross, D. R. (2007). *Counseling and psychotherapy: Theories and interventions* (4th ed.). New Jersey: Pearson Education Inc.

Corey, G. (1996). *Theory and practice of counseling and psychotherapy, enhanced* (10th ed.). Pacific Grove, CA: Brooks/Cole Publishing Company.

Corsini, R. J., & Wedding, D. (1995). *Current psychotherapies* (5th ed.). Itasca: F. E. Peacock Publishers Inc.

Frankl, V. E. (1992). Man's search for meaning: An introduction to logotherapy (4th ed.). Boston: Beacon Press.

Frankl, V. E. (2000). *Recollections: An autobiography.* New York: Basic Books.

Logotherapy. (2015, July 2). GoodTherapy. https://www.goodtherapy.org/learn-about-therapy/types/logotherapy#:~:text=The%20three%20main%20techniques%20of,about%20others%20rather%20than%20themselves

Pace, E. (1994, Oct 24). *Dr. Rollo May is dead at 85; Was innovator in psychology.* New York Times. Retrieved from http://search.proquest.com/docview/429909385?

Rollo May. (2015, July 20). GoodTherapy. https://www.goodtherapy.org/famous-psychologists/rollo-may.html

Vesely, F. J. (2020, April 10). *Viktor Frankl – bibliography.* https://www.viktorfrankl.org/biography.html#

Wedding, D., & Corsini, R. J. (2019). *Current psychotherapies* (11th ed.). Boston: Cengage Learning, Inc.

Yalom, I. (2017). *Becoming myself.* New York: Basic Books.

CONCLUSION: The End to the Real-Life Story of Donald Francis Kimball

Donny was an amazing young man with talent he could never really identify for himself. The world around him was in awe of his savant style abilities in all things mechanical. His charisma did not stop there. This red headed daredevil constantly drew crowds as he climbed heights that would have terrified a bystander. This ability to disregard his own safety led to his ability to commit suicide. With a house full of friends, he excused himself from the family room during a commercial break, went to his room, and took his own life.

His two sisters were sent to retrieve the neighborhood doctor while an ambulance was called. Because of the circumstances, CPR could be performed, the heart was kept beating, and when Donny arrived in the ER he was hooked up to extraordinary means. The hospital would now need two different EEGs, 24 hours apart from each other, in order to declare time of death.

As those hours ensued, the Church priest was called. At a time when organ donation was not a well-known procedure to the average person, the priest was asked by the hospital staff if he would be willing to approach the Kimballs about the possibility of donating Donny's organs. Although the church had no official stance at the time, the priest was more than willing to approach the family and support the idea, as it was life giving.

When the results of Donny's second EEG had come through and it was determined that he would be removed from life support, the Kimball's had been provided the time to decide that they did, indeed, believe in donating his organs. Once they agreed to the procedure, a team of surgeons from Stanford University Medical Center flew in to perform the surgery and remove his organs. They took his heart and kidneys.

As it turned out, a very close family friend was flying up to Stanford that night. He was a very spiritual man. As he was flying, he looked up and saw the stars, then looked down and saw the lights of the city below. He felt that God had cleared a safe path for Donny's heart to be flown to Stanford, so that it could provide life to another human being.

When this friend got to Stanford, he decided to drive to the hospital where Donny's heart would be giving life to another. When he got there, he found a woman and her three children sitting in the family waiting room. He asked the family if he could wait with them while the heart was being placed into her husband's chest. He identified himself as a friend of the donor's family. As they sat together, the recipient's wife described a hardworking, forty-two-year-old husband and father. She introduced this family friend to her children. She spoke about how this heart was not only restoring one life, but the life of an entire family. The donor family had touched so many more lives than they realized.

Suicide is an awful thing. It leaves family members and friends with a myriad of question for the rest of their lives. But this family was able to do something most suicide survivors are not able to do. They were able to donate their son's organs, and save the lives of others who were in need.

Donny's mother went on to become a transplant coordinator, one of the first. His father helped to start, in California, what was known as the pink card. This pink card was attached to a driver's license so that a hospital would know that you wanted to donate your organs in the midst of a crisis that had taken your life, should that day ever tragically and unexpectedly arrive.

The authors of this book have used the life of Donny to show prospective counselors, therapists, and psychologists what it is like to sit in a therapy session with a client and use a specific theoretical approach to guide a client into a place of hope. Although the ultimate ending to Donny's life was tragic, the many ways in which his death has furthered the field of transplantation, and will hopefully help students in their pursuit of a healing profession in the field of psychology, have helped his family find peace in an otherwise tragic situation.

APPENDICES

APPENDIX A: General Documents for Therapeutic Use

        Document 1: Confidentiality Agreement

        Document 2: Release of Information

        Document 3: Intake

        Document 4: Suicidal Risk Assessment

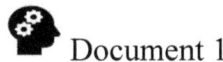 Document 1

Confidentiality Agreement

Confidentiality means that I, as the therapist, have a responsibility to safeguard information obtained during therapy. All information disclosed during a therapy session is kept confidential, except as mandated by law.

Limitations and Exceptions to Confidentiality: If you decide that you would like me to talk to someone about information provided during a session for the benefit of the therapeutic process, then you may sign a release of information allowing me to do so. Once the release is obtained then I may speak with someone on your behalf.

The Law requires me to disclose information in the following cases:

Suspected child or elder abuse
Potential harm to self or others
Information subpoenaed by a Court of Law

I have read the information provided to me regarding my confidentiality and the limitations to confidentiality. I fully understand the extent to which information must be provided by law and I agree to the terms of confidentiality.

Should my confidentiality be broken for legal reasons, I understand that I will be unable to take legal actions.

_____   _____

Printed Name   Signature

_____

Date

_____   _____

Witnesses Name   Witnesses Signature

_____

Date

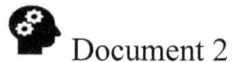 Document 2

Release of Information

Information Regarding the use of this disclosure:

I, _____, acknowledge that I am currently seeking therapy from this facility.

I hereby authorize the use of the information being released, including any protected health information discussed during my therapy sessions, as described below. Pursuant to 45 CFR 164.501 "Therapeutic Plan" refers to the plan created between the client and the therapist for the purpose of obtaining goals determined during the initial and ongoing therapeutic sessions. "Notes" refers to any form of documentation taken during a private therapy session whether done as an individual, joint, or family session and are separated from the rest of the individual's medical record.

For the purpose of improving my therapeutic experience, I authorize this facility and my therapist to obtain and provide information about my coaching session from and to:

_____

Organization's name (if applicable)

_____

Person's name to receive and release information to

_____

Address 1

_____

Address 2

_____

Phone

Information may be sent and received in the following manner:

_____E-mail   _____Phone   _____Mail   _____Text

_____In Person

The release allows the following information to be discussed either in person, by phone, or in writing:

_____Service Plan   _____Session Notes   _____Financial Information

Important information about your client rights:

I understand that this authorization is voluntary. I may refuse to sign it if I so wish.
I understand that this authorization is good for one year from the date of signature.
I understand that I may revoke this release at any time, but this facility and my therapist will not be held responsible for any information released prior to revocation of the release.
I understand that I will receive therapy sessions regardless of whether or not I sign this release.
I understand that my therapist and all employees that work for this facility are not responsible for how information is re-disclosed by parties to which the information has been disclosed.

Signature of Client and Witness:

_____
Printed Name of Client

_____   _____
Signature of Client   Date Signed

_____
Printed Name of Witness

_____   _____
Signature of Witness   Date Signed

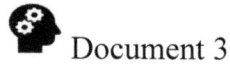 Document 3

Counseling Intake Form

Section 1: General Information

Name: _____   Date of Birth: _____

Age: _____   Gender: ___Male   ___Female   ___Other (identify)_____

Home Address: _____

Name of Employer or School: _____

Home phone: _____   Is it ok to phone? ___Yes ___No

May we leave a message? ___Yes   ___No

Cell phone: _____   Is it ok to phone? ___Yes ___No

May we leave a message? ___Yes   ___No

Work phone: _____   Is it ok to phone? ___Yes ___No

May we leave a message? ___Yes   ___No

Marital status: ___Never married ___Married ___Divorced ___Separated ___Widowed

Please list any children/age: _____

Section 2: General Health and Mental Health Information

How would you describe your current physical health? (circle one)

Poor   Unsatisfactory   Satisfactory   Good   Very Good

Please list any health problems you are currently experiencing:
_____
_____

Have you previous received any type of mental health services (e.g., psychotherapy, psychiatric services, etc.)? ___Yes   ___No

Previous therapist/practitioner: _____

Are you currently taking any prescription medication? ___Yes   ___No

Please list: _____

Please provide information about yourself or your child if you are a parent or guardian. This information will help better understand the problem you are having. The information is confidential and will not be released to anyone without your permission.

____ Depression   ____ Parent-child conflict   ____ Suicidal thoughts

____ Anxiety   ____ Panic attacks   ____ Suicidal actions

____ Anger/Temper   ____ Alcohol abuse   ____ Drug abuse

____ Job/School Problems   ____ Financial concerns   ____ Legal problems

____ Low self-esteem   ____ Relationship problems   ____ Medical problems

Other:_____

Please provide information about any of the following feelings that apply to you.

____ Angry   ____ Guilty   ____ Unhappy   ____ Bored   ____ Sad

____ Conflicted ____ Fearless ____ Happy   ____ Lonely   ____ Hopeless

____ Centered   ____ Fearful   ____ Excited   ____ Regretful ____ Anxious

____ Energetic ____ Content   ____ Envious   ____ Jealous ____ Other: _____

What issues/concerns have resulted in you seeking therapy at this time?
_____
_____
_____
_____
_____

What do you hope to gain from therapy?
_____
_____
_____
_____
_____

_____   _____
Name   Date

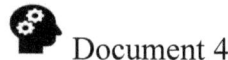 Document 4

Suicidal Risk Assessment

There are many factors that can contribute to the suicidality of a client. Regardless of why they are suicidal, it is important to gather information to determine if they simply want to fade into the background of life until things calm down? Or if they are actually thinking about committing suicide. The following questions will help you to determine the likelihood that they are in current need of hospitalization. This is not a form that you will hand your client. It is a form for you to start the conversation and determine how serious they are.

Do you feel hopeless about this situation?

Does this situation make you feel like hurting yourself?

How would you do that?

Are you considering taking your own life?

What makes you feel like you want to do that?

Have you made plans to do so?

How would you do it?

When were you planning to following through with it?

Has anyone in your family either attempted or completed a suicide?

How long ago?

What method did they use?

How did it make you feel when they did that?

Have any of your friends attempted suicide?

How long ago?

What method did they use?

How did it make you feel when they did that?

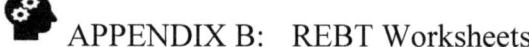 APPENDIX B: REBT Worksheets

    Document 1: A-B-C Model

    Document 2: Identifying Should, Must, and Need Thinking

    Document 3: Identifying the Root of Your Depression

    Document 4: SMART Goal Worksheet

    Document 5: Unhelpful Styles of Thinking

    Document 6: Identifying Maladaptive Thinking

    Document 7: De-catastrophizing

    Document 8: De-catastrophizing Worksheet

    Document 9: Rational VS Irrational Thinking (Fact or Opinion)

    Document 10: Putting Your Negative Thought on Trial

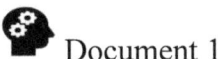
Document 1

A – B – C Model

A – An external or "activating" event

B – The interpretation or "belief" about the event

C – The "consequences" of our emotions & behavior

D – The "disputation" of an irrational belief

E – The "effect" or new belief as the result

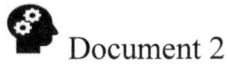 Document 2

Identifying Should, Must, and Need Thinking

Over the next week complete this form with one or more situations in your life that lead to a consequence you are uncomfortable with. Then bring it back to your next therapy session.

1) Describe a situation that led to undesired consequences:

2) Describe the undesired consequence:

3) Label the undesired emotion you feel about the occurrence and rate it on a scale of 1-10:

4) What do you think should have happened, needed to happen, or must happen in relation to this situation?

5) Can you restate that thought without the words should, must, or need?

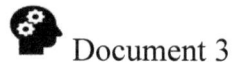 Document 3

Identifying the Root of Your Depression

Please give a brief description of what you think is the reason for your depression:

Is there substantial evidence for that thought process?

_____Yes _____No

List your evidence:

Is there substantial evidence to the contrary?

_____Yes _____No

List your evidence:

Will the situation that has led to your depression matter in 6 months? Explain.

Will it matter in 1 year?

Are you attempting to interpret the reason you are depressed without all the evidence?

_____Yes _____No

Describe why you think this?

Depression most often stems from 3 irrational thought patterns:
1. Self-Blame –
2. Self-Pity –
3. Other Pity –

Given the above information are you now able to identify the root of your depression from the list above?

_____Yes   _____No

If so, which root cause appears to be the root of your depression?

Does knowing the above information change your belief on why you are depressed?

How?

If you had to describe why you are depressed at this point in the exercise what would you say?

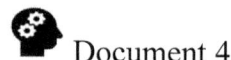 Document 4

SMART Goal Worksheet

Answer the questions below to help you write a concise and specific goal

What are you trying to accomplish?_____
_____
_____
_____

S stands for Specific. What are the specifics of your goal? Answer the following questions.

Who will be part of accomplishing this goal?_____
_____
_____
_____

What is required to accomplish this goal?_____
_____
_____
_____

Where will this goal be accomplished? (Work, home, school, etc...)_____
_____
_____
_____

Why do I want to accomplish this goal?   _____
_____
_____
_____

When will I be accomplishing this goal? (Now, next week, over the next year)_____
_____
_____
_____

M stands for Measurable. How will you measure whether or not you have accomplished this goal? For instance, will an application be printed, completed, or turned in?

What is the specific way in which you are going to measure the accomplishment of this goal?___
_____
_____
_____

A stands for Attainable. What resources in my environment will allow me to attain this goal?

What resources are necessary to accomplish this goal?_____
_____
_____
_____

Do I have access to those resources?_____
_____
_____
_____

If not, then is there a way to make those resources available?_____
_____
_____
_____

Is this goal attainable?   Yes____   No____

R stands for Realistic. The resources are available and I can attain this goal at this time. Is it realistic?

Do I have the time to accomplish this goal?   Yes____   No____

How will accomplishing this goal affect me?_____
_____
_____
_____

How will accomplishing this goal affect those around me?_____
_____
_____
_____

Is this goal realistic?   Yes____   No____

T stands for Time-bound. When will this goal be accomplished by?

Is there a specific due date for this goal already set by an external entity?   Yes___   No___

If yes, when is that due date?_____

If no, when do you think the earliest time is that you could accomplish the tasks required to accomplish this goal?_____

Are there things that might get in the way of you accomplishing this goal by the above date?

Yes___   No___

What might get in your way?_____
_____
_____
_____

If yes, is it realistic to move the date out a few days or a week?   Yes___   No___

What is the final decision on the date you will accomplish this goal?_____
_____
_____

With all the information above it is time to rewrite your goal using the above information.

My goal is:_____
_____
_____
_____

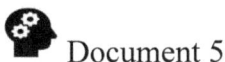 Document 5

Unhelpful Styles of Thinking

Awfulizing

Personalization

(Maladaptive Thought Processes)

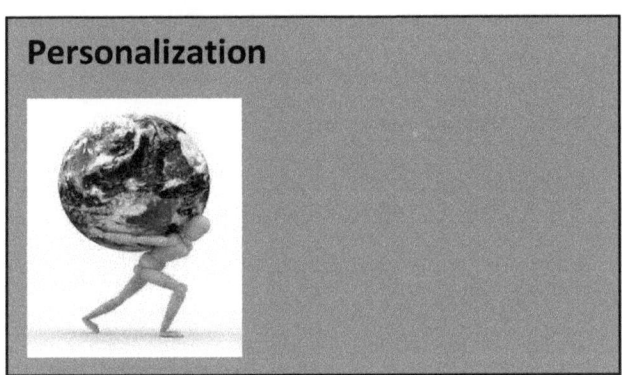

Overgeneralizing

Drawing a conclusion from a single, negative event.

Nothing is ever good.

Always
Never
All of Them
None of Them
Everybody
Nobody
All of the
None of th

Taking responsibility for something that is not your fault.

Assuming the

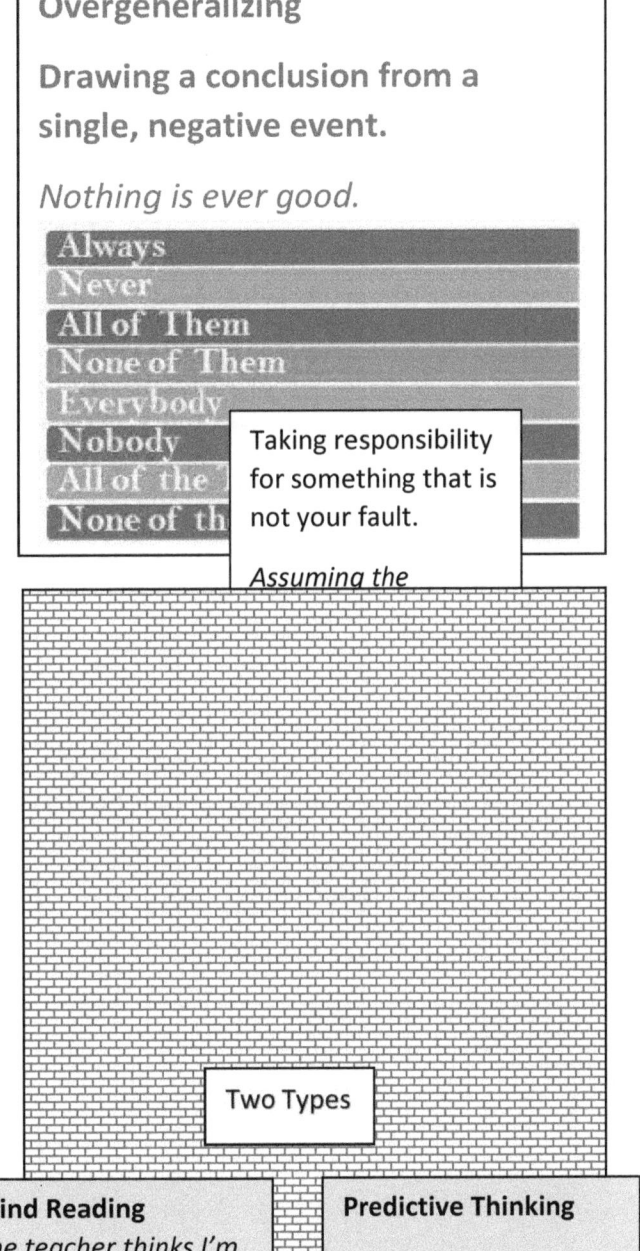

Jumping

Assuming w evidence.

Fact

Imagining that a situation is worse than it really is.

If you fail a test, you are a failure.

Two Types

Mind Reading
The teacher thinks I'm stupid because I didn't know the answer.

Predictive Thinking
No one will come to my birthday party.

Should Statements – putting unreasonable demands on yourself.

"I should always be happy"

out of proportion.

Minimization – Making a situation seem less important.

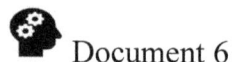

Identifying Maladaptive Thinking

Every person on this Earth suffers from cognitive distortions at one time or another. They are a normal part of the human condition. However, when we put too much weight on thinking that is over influenced by cognitive distortion, or we only see the world through a specific cognitive distortion, then our understanding of a situation can become skewed. It can affect our interpersonal relationships, as well as the decisions that we make every day.

Below are common distortions that occur in our thoughts from time-to-time. Take a few minutes to read about each distortion. Then write down one time that you remember utilizing each one. There may be a few distortions that you don't have an example for. Don't worry, just move on to the next description. Finally, determine if there are any distortions that you use on a regular basis. If there are, then it would be beneficial for you to work on and challenge this pattern of thinking.

1) All-or-Nothing Thinking/ Polarized Thinking

When someone engaged in All-or-Nothing thinking, they tend to see the world as very black and white. Things are either good or bad, right or wrong, or positive or negative. There is no continuum for this kind of thinking, no shades of gray in a situation.

Personal example:
_____
_____

2) Overgeneralization

This occurs when we take one occurrence or situation, and assume that all incidences that follow will be the same. For instance, that one roller coaster broke down while I was on it, therefore all roller coasters will break down while I am on them. A more common way that this often plays out is, that person betrayed me, therefore all people will betray me. This leads to negative perceptions about the world around us, and can often lead to negative emotions about the world and our place in it.

Personal example:
_____
_____

3) Mental Filter

A mental filter occurs when a person looks at an event and only sees the negative things that have happened. They do not look at an event as a whole. For instance, the person may have had friends over, it was a wonderful event, but someone made a sarcastic comment. The only thing the person thinks about is the comment, and it ruins the whole evening for them. Why? Because they are not focusing on all the fun that was had, only on the one bad comment. When this is a predominant way of thinking, you can become pessimistic about the world.

Personal example:
_____
_____

4) Disqualifying the Positive

This distortion is a little bit different than the mental filter. This person will recognize that something positive has happened to them. They simply don't give the positive thing any weight. For example, a person in college gets an A on their report card, but instead of acknowledging all the hard work they put into it, they say it is because the professor feels sorry for them.

Personal example:
_____
_____

5) Mind Reading

Mind reading is the belief that you know what another person is thinking. For instance, they may have a friend who is having a bad day. This person has a sour look on their face, or a brooding tone of voice. Because of this, they decide that their friend hates them. In this instance, they are jumping to a false conclusion, that they believe with all their heart is correct.

Personal example:

_____
_____

6) Fortune Telling

When someone exhibits Fortune Telling, they have a tendency to draw conclusions about the future without any real evidence. The predictions are negative in nature. The person with this tendency treats their predictions as fact. One example of this is that a person in their late 20's might decide that because they aren't married yet, they are never going to have children. They are drawing this conclusion based on their age. But evidence does not support this.

Personal example:

_____
_____

7) Catastrophizing

When someone catastrophizes, they take an event and make it more dramatic than it really is. For instance, a person may get injured and feel pain. But instead of focusing on the healing process, they focus on the pain and are convinced that it will get worse and prevent them from doing things that they want to for the rest of their life.

Personal example:

_____
_____

8) Minimizing

When a person minimizes, they are taking something big and acting as if it is no big deal. For instance, a person who has cancer may say it is not a big deal, they will just go through the treatment and be all better.

Personal example:

_____
_____

9) Emotional Reasoning

Emotional Reasoning occurs when a person believes that because they feel something, it must be true. For instance, a person may feel jealous and believe that a co-worker is hitting on their spouse, and trying to break up their marriage. They believe this to be utterly true. But there may be absolutely no fact in what the spouse thinks. In fact, the other person may be happily married.

Personal example:

_____
_____

10) Should Statements

Should Statements use words such as should, ought, and must. They are all or nothing statements that impose strict expectations of ourselves and others. When we convince ourself of the should statements, and we do not live up to the expectations that they set, it is common to feel guilt. When others do not live up to the should and ought statements that we believe, we are often stuck with a feeling of disappointment. This can lead to resentment of another person.

Personal example:

_____
_____

11) Labeling and Mislabeling

We label or mislabel when we have one experience and we assign a judgment of value to either ourself or someone else. For instance, we may fall once in public and label ourself a klutz. Or another person might be having a bad day and yell at us, and we mislabel them as mean and nasty.

Personal example:
_____
_____

12) Personalization

This distortion occurs when you assume that things are connected to you, even when they are not. For instance, you might believe that your child is struggling in school because you did something wrong as a parent.

Personal example:
_____
_____

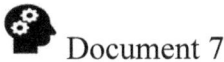 Document 7

De-catastrophizing

What is the current problem that is bothering you?

How likely is it that the problem will occur?

1   2   3   4   5   (1 unlikely – 5 likely)

If the problem does take place, what is the worst thing that could happen?

Provide Evidence (has this happened before?)

If this problem does take place, what is the best-case scenario?

What coping strategies could you use if this problem does occur?

If the problem does occur, what are the chances you will be ok?

___% in a week   ___% in a month   ___%in a year

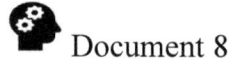 Document 8

De-catastrophizing Worksheet

Thoughts very often influence how a person feels. When these thoughts are irrational, they can bring up very strong feelings about something. These strong feelings can make the situation feel overwhelming. When we feel overwhelmed, it can become difficult to make good choices.

Once common cognitive distortion is called catastrophizing. This happens when we think of a situation and then either exaggerate our thinking about it, or we assume that the worst possible outcome will occur.

One way to manage such reactions to our thoughts and fears, is to question them in a logical way. This helps us determine if our thoughts are based on many experiences and facts, or if one bad experience or fact has been blown out of proportion to facilitate a cognitive distortion. This worksheet will help you to determine if you are catastrophizing a specific situation in your life.

Write down what you are worried about.

On a scale of 1-10, how anxious are you about the situation?

__1   __2   __3   __4   __5   __6   __7   __8   __9   __10

How likely is it that you fear about this situation will come true?

What past experiences have helped you to form this concern?

What is the supporting evidence that your anxiety about this situation is valid?

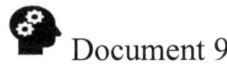 Document 9

Rational VS Irrational Thinking
Fact or Opinion

To understand rational vs irrational thinking, it is helpful to think about your thoughts as fact or opinion. A fact is verifiable. It has supporting information to back it up. Opinions, on the other hand, come from our personal interpretation of the facts. It can take some practice to separate the two out. Let's use food to create an example. We are eating friend chicken tonight is a fact. The fried chicken tastes good tonight is an opinion.

The example above is clear and easy to pull apart. But sometimes we impose irrational thinking on ourselves or others and view it is fact. For instance, an attractive person might think to themselves "I am ugly." The brain might see this as fact. But beauty is in the eye of the beholder. It is an opinion, and in this case, it is an irrational thought.

Below you will find some examples of rational thinking and some examples of irrational thinking. Put an X in the column that fits the statement.

The thought	Rational/Fact	Irrational/Opinion
I have a blemish on my face		
I am a good artist		
Borgo Italia is a great restaurant		
Pancakes are made with flour		
I didn't get my homework done because I needed to talk to Jane		
That movie was so scarry!		
My teacher is so mean!		
My Science Teacher worked at NASA		
I broke my arm falling out of a tree.		

Now it is your turn. Over the next few days, take time to write down some of the thoughts that run through your head. Don't worry about how you think they will be perceived by others. The thoughts you have affect the way you behave, so it is important to identify what those thoughts are.

Once you are satisfied with your list, sit down and determine which of your thoughts are rational, and which are irrational. As you continue to practice this skill, you will become better at challenging your irrational thoughts. Overtime, rational thoughts will begin to immerge naturally.

There are many spaces for you to write down your thoughts. You do not need to fill in every line. Just write down thoughts as they come to you, and when the sheet is available at your fingertips. When you have several boxes completed, sit down and determine which thoughts are rational, and which ones are not. If you want to feel in each space, then don't try to do it all at once. Simply do the sheet over several weeks.

The thought	Rational/Fact	Irrational/Opinion

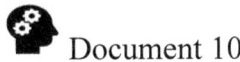 Document 10

Putting Your Negative Thought on Trial

This technique is used to determine if the negative thought you are having is helpful or harmful. Some negative thoughts have value. They warn us not to make a bad decision. They keep us from re-engaging in unhealthy relationships. Most negative thoughts, however, are a product of distorted thinking, that often times leads to unhealthy decision making.

On the next page, you are being provided with a space to write out your negative thought. You will also notice a box labeled judge, prosecution, and defense. In the box marked prosecution, write down all supporting evidence that this thought might **NOT** be true or helpful. The prosecution is trying to prove the thought wrong. In the defense box, write down all the supporting evidence that this thought might **BE** true or helpful. This defense is trying to state that the thought is necessary and true. Once you have gone through that process, evaluate both sides of the evidence. Take time to determine whether the thought is helpful or not. If it is helpful for your life, then write innocent in the judge's box. If the thought is unhelpful, write guilty in that box.

You can take this one step further if you so desire. If the verdict is guilty, it can be helpful to tear the sheet up into little pieces to let your brain recognize that it does not need this thought.

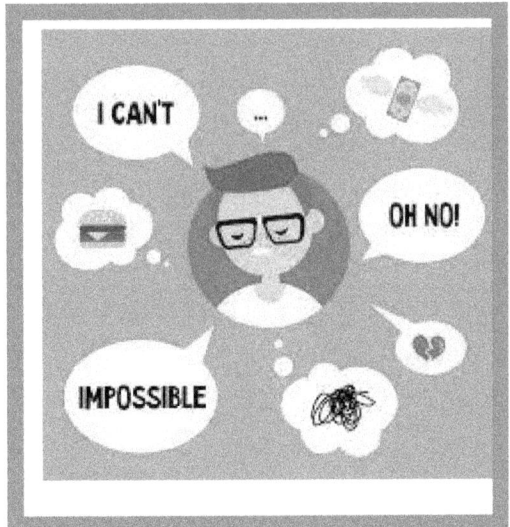

Putting Your Negative Thought on Trial

Negative thought:
_____
_____
_____

Judge	
Prosecution	**Defense**

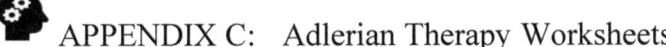APPENDIX C: Adlerian Therapy Worksheets

        Document 1: Lifestyle Questionnaire – Family Constellation

        Document 2: Lifestyle Questionnaire – Dreams

        Document 3: Lifestyle Questionnaire – Early Recollections

        Document 4: Lifestyle Questionnaire – Social Interest

        Document 5: Push Button Technique

        Document 6: Reflecting As If VS Acting As If

        Document 7: Catching Oneself

        Document 8: Spitting in the Client's Soup

        Document 9: The Question

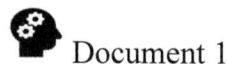 Document 1

Lifestyle Questionnaire – Family Constellation

Tell me about your family
_____
_____
_____
_____

Discuss your family values and their impact on your life
_____
_____
_____
_____
_____

Tell me about your relationship with your parents
_____
_____
_____
_____
_____

Who is most like your mother? Why?
_____
_____

Who is most like your father? Why?
_____
_____

Who is the family favorite? Why?
_____
_____

Siblings (name and age)

1._____   _____
2._____   _____
3._____   _____
4._____   _____

Family Characteristics (indicate family memory who displays these characteristics)

Intelligent_____	Most Fun Loving_____
Achievement oriented_____	Most Humorous_____
Hard Working_____	Most Easy Going_____
Family Favorite_____	Rule Follower_____
Most Needy_____	Athletic_____
Assertive_____	Rebellious_____
Charming_____	Spoiled_____
Critical of Others_____	Patient_____
Responsible_____	Imaginative_____
Materialistic_____	Lowest Self-Esteem_____
Withdrawn_____	Angry_____
Selfish_____	Talkative_____

Which sibling is the most different from you? How?
_____
_____
_____

Which sibling is the most similar to you? How?
_____
_____
_____

List interest or skills for each sibling

1._____
2._____
3._____
4._____

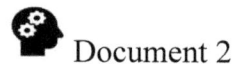 Document 2

Lifestyle Questionnaire – Dreams

Do you remember your dreams?   _____Yes   _____No

What is the first dream you remember having?
_____
_____
_____
_____

Do you have any reoccurring dreams?
_____
_____
_____
_____

Did you or do you presently suffer from nightmares? If so, what were they about?
_____
_____
_____
_____

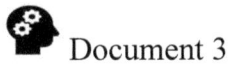 Document 3

Lifestyle Questionnaire – Early Recollections

Early Recollections

What is the first childhood memory that comes to mind?

_____
_____
_____
_____

What is your earliest childhood memory?

_____
_____
_____
_____

Were these positive or negative memories? Why?

_____
_____
_____
_____

Childhood

What were your strengths as a child?

_____
_____

What were your weaknesses as a child?

_____
_____

Who were your childhood friends? What did you do together?

1._____   3._____

2._____   4._____

_____
_____
_____

What were your childhood fears?

_____
_____
_____

What afterschool activities did you participate in?

_____
_____
_____

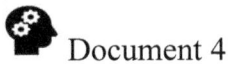
Document 4

Lifestyle Questionnaire – Social Interest

What are your hobbies?
_____
_____
_____
_____

What activities do you enjoy doing in your spare time?

____Reading	____Watching TV	____social media
____Writing	____Gaming	____Decorating
____Jogging	____Art	____Collecting
____Baking	____Crafts	____Making Music
____Refinishing Furniture	____Walking	____Sports
____Fostering animals	____DIY Projects	____Volunteering

Other:
_____
_____

How often do you feel positively about yourself? (circle on)

Never   Sometimes   Often   Almost Always

Are you sensitive to criticism? (circle one)

Never   Sometimes   Often   Almost Always

What do you feel is your best quality? _____

What do you feel is your worst quality? _____

Do you have any close friends? _____ If so, how frequently do you see them? _____

What's the quality of your relationship?
_____
_____
_____

Are you having issues with any specific person in your life? _____

What are the specific issues that are concerning you?
_____
_____
_____
_____

Do you have a job? _____ If so, where do you work? _____

What do you do?
_____
_____

What are your favorite things about your job?
_____
_____

What do you like least about your job?
_____
_____

Does your job provide any meaning in your life? _____ If so, explain
_____
_____
_____

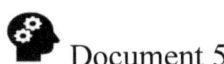 Document 5

PUSH BUTTON TECHNIQUE

Goal: To help clients understand their role in creating and sustaining unpleasant feelings.

STEP 1 — Recall a pleasant memory. Provide details about the memory. Focus on the positive feelings.

_____
_____
_____
_____
_____

STEP 2

Recall an unpleasant memory. Provide details about the memory. Focus on the negative feelings.

_____
_____
_____
_____
_____

STEP 3

Generate a new happy memory **OR** return to the happy memory from Step 1. Focus on positive feelings.

_____
_____
_____
_____
_____

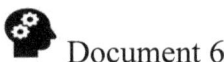 Document 6

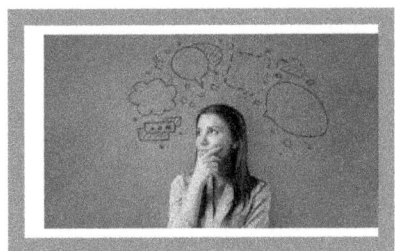

Reflecting As If
VS
Acting As If
Two Sides to the Same Coin

Often times, when a client feels as if they do not have a skill that they would like to obtain, these two techniques will facilitate the desired change that the client is looking for.

For instance, let's say a client does not feel confident. They watch their parent go out into public and exude confidence in their interactions. But the client feels shy and pulls away from social situations.

The first course of action for some therapists is to have the client

Reflect As IF

You can have a client close their eyes and imagine a specific scenario where they are behaving as confident as their mother.

- Ask them what they would say in that situation.
- Find out how they feel when they are exuding such confidence.
- Find out how their life would change if they behaved in life how they are behaving in this imagined scenario.

Once a client has gained some confidence in Reflecting As If, it is sometimes helpful to then challenge them to

Act As IF

Have the client pick a scenario in their life where they will act as if they have confidence. When they return for their session find out how it went?

- What did they like about approaching a situation with confidence? What was uncomfortable for them?
- How did things play out differently because they were not acting shy and withdrawing?
- If this is indeed a change that they would like to make in their life, have the repeat the assignment many times, in several different scenarios, until it becomes comfortable for them to act this way.

When clients are able to follow through on both these techniques, they often find themselves making the kinds of changes that promote physical and mental well-being in their life.

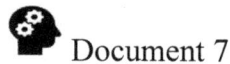 Document 7

Catching Oneself

This refers to a technique where patients 'catch themselves' performing behavior that they wish to change. By performing this technique, the client is becoming aware of and changing their own thoughts, feelings, and behaviors.

Negative Self-Talk

<u>Example</u>: I'm stupid, I don't know anything. Someone engaged in this type of negative self-talk may 'catch themselves' when starting to think or say something critical or self-deprecating. To challenge these negative thoughts replace them with more positive thoughts or ideas.

Personal Example:
_____
_____
_____

How Frequently does this behavior occur:

_____multiple times daily   _____once daily   _____multiple times a week

_____weekly   _____monthly   _____infrequently

Replacement Thought:
_____
_____
_____

How often have I caught myself engaging in negative self-talk?

Did I use my replacement thought when this occurred?

Was it effective?

Impulsive Behavior

Example: Yelling out an answer during a lecture. Someone engaged in impulsive behavior may 'catch themselves' in the act and think before proceeding. They might start to think of the consequences of their actions and make more thoughtful choices.

Personal Example:

_____
_____
_____

How Frequently does this behavior occur:

_____ multiple times daily _____ once daily _____ multiple times a week

_____ weekly _____ monthly _____ infrequently

Replacement Thought or Action:

_____
_____
_____

How often have I caught myself engaging in impulsive behavior?

Did I use my replacement thought/action when this occurred?

Was it effective?

Emotional Regulation

Example: Becoming overly anxious about an exam. Starting to be overwhelmed by everyday life. Someone who struggles with emotional regulation may 'catch themselves' when they are starting to become overwhelmed by these emotions. Using coping techniques (e.g., deep breathing, drawing) can help them manage their feelings in a more adaptive manner.

Personal Example:

_____
_____
_____

How Frequently does this behavior occur:

_____multiple times daily _____once daily _____multiple times a week

_____weekly _____monthly _____infrequently

Replacement Thought or Action:
_____
_____
_____

How often have I caught myself engaging in impulsive behavior?

Did I use my replacement thought/action when this occurred?

Was it effective?

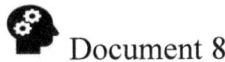 Document 8

Spitting in the Client's Soup

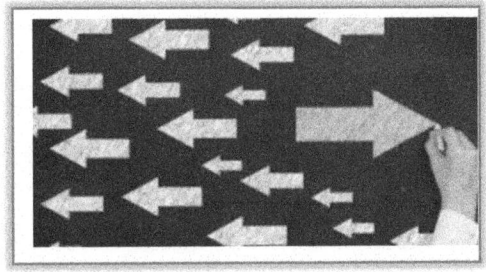

This is a useful strategy for client's who avoid the demands and/or responsibilities of life. Spitting in the Client's Soup is a metaphor for destroying the avoidance strategy.

Example: A client comes to the therapist feeling frustrated with being the only one to take care of the household chores. She feels undervalued by her family and is frequently run down. The therapist may say: it's ok if you are constantly run down and sick. This is the only time you are able to be taken care of by others. You are affirming that the needs of your client are not being met.

This Spitting in the Client's Soup worksheet will help the client explore how they are sabotaging their own success and provide insight into the meaning of their behavior and how to improve their own well-being.

Spitting in the Client's Soup

Describe a negative behavior that is harmful towards yourself or others?	
What is the intention behind the behavior?	
What are the benefits of this behavior?	
What are the consequences of this behavior?	
Is there a healthier replacement behavior you could put into place?	
How can the replacement behavior be more productive?	

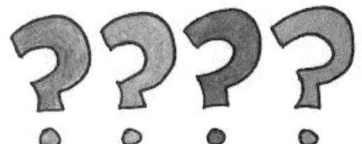
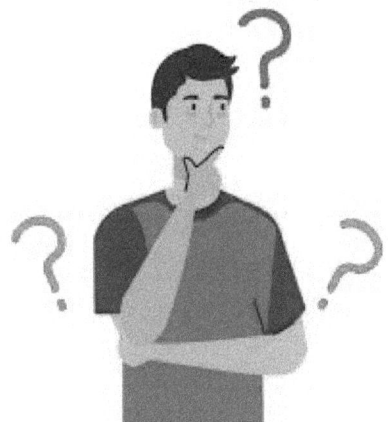

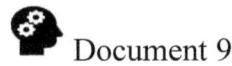 Document 9

The Question

Alfred Adler noticed that sometimes patients focused too much on their own experience. This egotistic view that they were stuck in, often kept them from being able to see alternative views of their situation. One way to move the client from the egocentric view that was disturbing them, was to ask a question that moved their focus to other.

To do that, Alfred Adler would ask this question:

If you had a magic wand, and the problem you just described was solved with the wave of it, how would your life change?

Other Adlerians have been known to pose the question another way:

What negative consequences might ensue for those around you if you could wave a magic wand and make this situation go away?

Or also:

How would your life be different if you did not have (the therapist then names a symptom)?

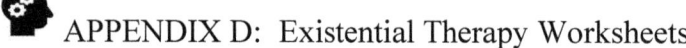 APPENDIX D: Existential Therapy Worksheets

                     Document 1: The Empty Chair Technique

                     Document 2: De-reflection Exercise

                     Document 3: De-reflection Worksheet

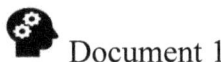 Document 1

The Empty Chair Technique

The empty chair technique in Existential Therapy is used when someone has trepidation about how a conversation might go. It can be a conversation with a boss, a co-worker or even a loved one. Often, the fear the client has about the conversation, prevents them from starting the conversation in the first place, but once they "play out" how the conversation might go, they gain the confidence to follow through with it.

As the therapist you will place two chairs, facing each other. Ask the client to sit in a chair. Once they are seated, this chair will represent them self. The other chair, will represent the person that they are speaking with.

Let the client know that they will be working through a possible way that the conversation might go, using the two chairs. When they are sitting in the chair they are in now, they will "play" the role of them self. When they are sitting in the opposite chair, they will "play" the role of the person they are preparing to have a conversation with.

Have the client start the conversation as them self. When they are finished with what they have to say, have them get up, go to the other chair, and sit back down. Once they are in that chair, have them respond as if they were the other person. They will go back and forth like this until the conversation is complete.

Once the conversation is complete, review the conversation with the client. What went the way they had preconceived it before they "played" the opposite person. What went the way that they expected? What was different? Has this changed the level of anxiety that they feel about having the conversation? Has this information changed the way that they intend to approach the conversation? If so, how? If so, would they like to do the technique again, to find out how it will change?

THE PROCESS

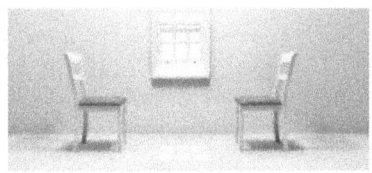

First: Pretend there is a person sitting in front of you.

-What is the person's name?

-It could be an aspect of yourself, such as anger.

Second: Begin speaking to this person/thing as if it was directly in front of you seated in the chair.

Third: Move to the empty chair. Take a deep breath and become that person/thing. Bring qualities of that person/thing to your mind. Then respond to what was just heard from "you" sitting in the oppositive chair.

Fourth: Move back to the original chair. Breath again and discuss what was just said.

Fifth: Breath again and reflect on the experience.

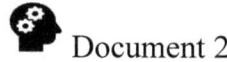 Document 2

De-reflection Exercise

Existential Therapists often utilize de-reflection during a session. It is the process of interrupting a client who is overly focused on them self, and moving the attention elsewhere. Keep in mind that this is done genuinely and with compassion. This is not a technique to be used with a narcissistic client. Patients often become overly focused on themselves when they have been hurt, or there is a struggle for which they have no control over. By learning to remove the focus from themselves, you are teaching them a coping skill to reduce their anxiety and improve their ability to have compassion for others.

At one point in the book this was used with Donny when we moved the focus from himself, to the possible realities of the teacher that he did not get along with. Instead of only viewing his relationship with this teacher though the eyes of his disability, he was asked to consider whether the teacher had ever worked with a student who had an IEP. The goal, is to help the client become well rounded in their view of the world around them.

The following homework sheet is designed for the therapist to send home with the client after they have used the technique in sessions with them. It requires that the therapist explain that the purpose of this worksheet is to help them see a situation from all sides, not to judge their behavior in the situation. The goal here is not for the client to go home and beat themselves up after they have completed the exercise, but to allow them to see the situation from every direction.

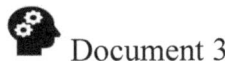 Document 3

De-reflection Worksheet

Just as we look in a mirror and focus on the first thing that we see, we tend to overfocus on situations that are occurring, and spend too much time thinking about them only from our own perspective. Just as it is more healthy to move your focus off of the blemish in the mirror, and on to other parts of your face, we want to move the focus in a situation off of yourself and onto the others who are also involved in the situation. The purpose is to ensure that you have a well-rounded view of what is going on.

Write down an example of a situation that has either hurt or offended you
Example:

List the names of People involved in this situation. Under their name write down their reaction to the situation
Name(s) and Reaction(s):

Pick one person out of the list of people above, close your eyes, and imagine the situation through their eyes. Sit with what you imagine to be their perspective of the situation for a bit. How do you imagine that they felt at the time? What might have been their possible motivation for the way that they acted? Are you aware of anything in their past that might have made the situation hurtful or offensive to them? Are there relevant facts worth observing about that person's life which would put their attitude into perspective for you?

Perspective of those involved in the situation (how they felt, motivation, etc.):

Now that you have completed this exercise, what have you learned from it? Did you gain any peace from this exercise? Did you gain any compassion for that person that you did not have before? Are there things that you would do differently if that situation were to present itself again? In the blanks space below, write down any insight that you gained from looking at the situation from all sides.

Insight(s):

Acknowledgements

We would like to thank the Kimball Family for allowing us to use Donny's story. It has allowed us to honor him in both life and death. We are so grateful to his parents, Lee and Gerry, for providing us with all the documentation that they had collected over the years, and for sharing his story with us each time that we reached out. We are also grateful to Joanne and Susan for sharing their memories along the journey of this book.

About The Authors

Joanne received her B.A. degree in Psychology from Saint Mary's College of California in 1995. After working for a year post graduation, she enrolled in graduate school at Marymount University in Arlington, Virginia where she received her Master's of Arts in Counseling Psychology. After working many years as a therapist, Joanne took some time off when her daughter was born. Upon returning to work she decided to pursue a career in Mental Health Life Coaching. Joanne is now a Board-Certified Coach.

Jessica received her B.S. degree in Psychology from Pennsylvania State University in 2002. After working in Washington, DC for a few years following graduation, she decided to enroll in graduate school at Georgia State University. While at Georgia State, she co-authored a number of journal articles related to neuropsychology, multiculturalism, data-based decision making, and mindfulness. Jessica earned a M.Ed., Ed.S., and Ph.D. in School Psychology. Jessica has been employed as a school psychologist in Georgia for 17 years. Currently, she resides in Peachtree City, GA with her husband and three children.